THE
PLANT
POWER
DOCTOR

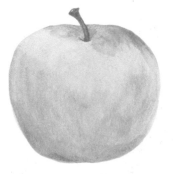

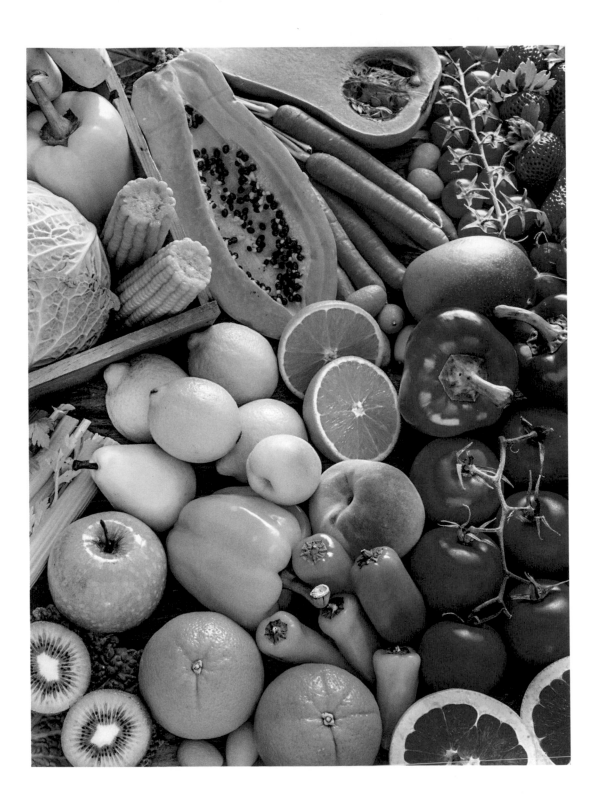

THE
PLANT
POWER
DOCTOR

A simple
prescription for
a healthier you

Dr Gemma Newman

EBURY
PRESS

CONTENTS

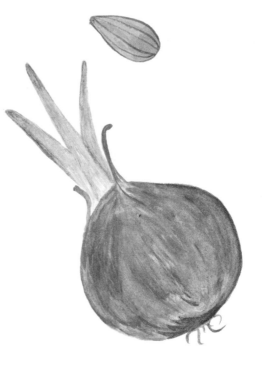

INTRODUCTION

If there was one simple change you could make to your lifestyle that would offer remarkable benefits for your physical and mental health, reducing your risk of many diseases and boosting your mood and well-being, while also helping the environment, would you like to know more?

It is very easy when you know how:

EAT MORE PLANTS

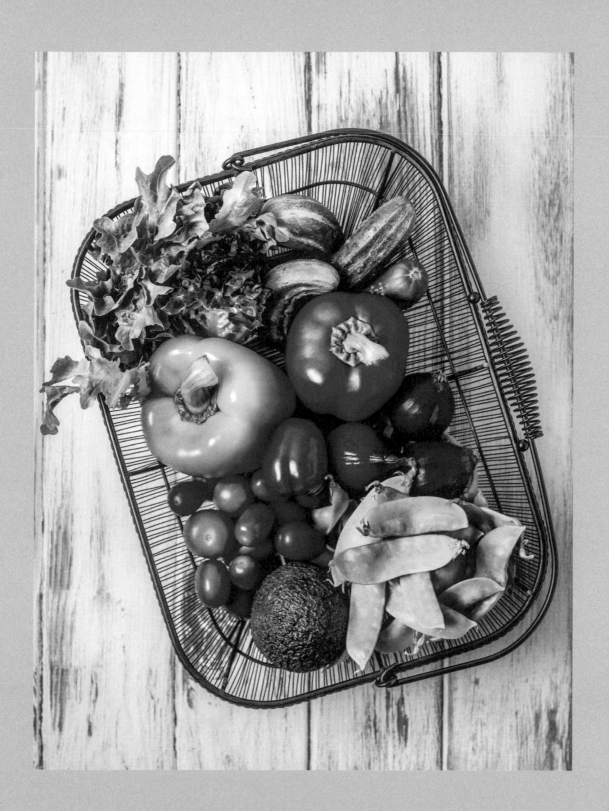

My name is Gemma and I have been a doctor for 17 years. Like most doctors, I went into my career with the aim of wanting to help people. I chose to become a GP because I love getting to know people, their families, the communities in which they live, and being by their side from cradle to grave. A friend once described Family Medicine to me as the branch of medicine where we get to 'save lives in slow motion' and I think this sums it up perfectly. My ten-minute appointment time goes by in a flash; as well as diagnosing and treating illnesses, I aim to use this time to help my patients change their lives for the better. In the modern age, a time when communities and family links are becoming so rare, people come to the doctor for so much more than medical advice. They seek a friend, a confidante, a counsellor, and sometimes everything all at once. People let me into their lives and trust me and for that, I feel hugely privileged.

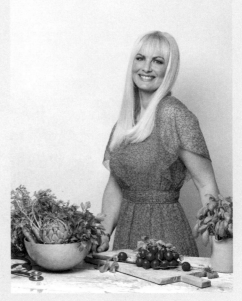

Over the years I have grown to understand how wonderful – and yet how limited – the medical model can be. When we have a car accident and need emergency surgery, or when we need a life-saving course of antibiotics for sepsis, the advances we have made in modern medicine are nothing short of extraordinary. But chronic diseases like back pain, depression, diabetes and heart disease? Treating them is much harder. Helping people deal with their diseases without a magic wand is a really difficult thing to do. In my profession, there are many patterns, guidelines, and templates in place to 'fix' people and the question of 'what' often becomes more important than the 'why'. For me, the question 'why is this person suffering?' is far more important than 'what is the diagnosis?'

When I first started work as a doctor, I realised that while I had plenty of information and knowledge in my toolbox, it was still half empty. On many occasions, no matter how many packets of tablets or procedures I offered my patients, I was left with the unshakeable feeling that I had not helped them. Side effects and interactions of a variety of medicines – especially in my elderly patients – could sometimes do more harm than good.

I couldn't help but wonder if there was a better way.

I continued to study. I researched psychology, lifestyle medicine and ideas of holistic medicine. This is a form of medical care that looks at the whole person and how all aspects of their life are balanced, with the aim of not just finding a diagnosis and forming a treatment plan, but also noticing what may have led to that diagnosis. When someone is living with a chronic disease, it's much trickier to understand why a symptom has arisen but it's central to true healing. What food does a person eat? Who are they surrounded by? What do they do for a living? What is their social life like? How well do they sleep at night? All these questions are key when fitting the puzzle pieces of the 'why' of disease into a picture we can recognise.

Medical training, by necessity, sometimes forces you to close your mind to the unknown. We are taught to be specific, to look for solid outcomes and to follow the evidence base. With all this structure and security, it can make a doctor feel very inadequate when their patient doesn't fit the box, and if their symptoms don't go away. So, I have had to look outside the diagnostic boxes I was taught to put people in and I made it my mission to be open to new ideas. I learned more about psychological interventions; ways I could support people change their mindset to facilitate change or growth, or to help them with their mental health, and I always wondered if there was a formula that could allow for true health and healing.

A CHANCE DISCOVERY

My journey to plant-based advocacy came about by chance. Several ago, my husband Richard was training to run the London Marathon and he was getting injury after injury with inflamed hips and ankles. Hobbling home after yet another thwarted training run, he was disappointed and wanted to be well enough to do his best, so he started looking into ways to help himself. He started to read about what ultra-runners do – how did they manage to run for hundreds of miles at a time? He soon found that many of these runners had something in common: they ate a wholefoods plant-based diet.

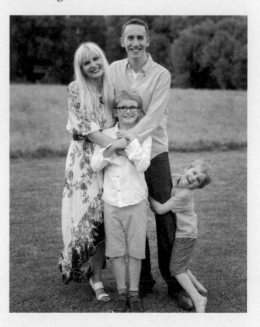

'I'm going to give it a try,' he said to me one night. I had never looked into plant-based diets before and to be honest, my first instinct was one of horror: 'What will our friends say? We'll be social outcasts! How are you supposed to get enough protein?!' I had a suspicion that these athletes' successes were more likely rooted in their technique than their food. But more importantly: Who would I share my favourite Friday night steak and chips with now?

Richard started eating more beans, rice, vegetables and fruit, and stopped eating meat, dairy, eggs, refined flour or sugar. He made huge progress with his training and stopped getting injured. He was training less and making better times. His inflamed ankles returned to normal. He could run a marathon before breakfast then look after the kids all day! I figured this must be some sort of coincidence but then I looked into the medical literature. The evidence for increasing the proportion of whole plant foods was compelling and persuasive. I felt quite embarrassed for being so sure that food had nothing to do with it; I could see the changes were really beneficial for him. I began to realise that my husband, who is not a medic, was teaching me something really valuable that I could add to my medical practice.

We grew up knowing that eating vegetables was a good thing, but not how good, or how transformative a plant-based diet could be. Why wasn't the message being spread more widely? Within six months on a wholefoods plant-based diet, Richard ran the marathon again, 1 hour and 10 minutes faster than his first attempt.

MY OWN HEALTH JOURNEY

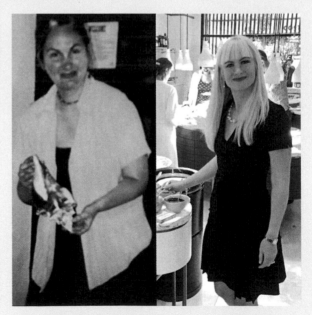

As a young doctor in a high-pressure environment, like many new physicians, I often neglected my own health. I ate too much of the wrong kinds of foods, I often felt tired and my BMI was not in the healthy range. I wanted to feel better and have more energy to do my job. And I felt like a hypocrite. How could I tell people how to be healthier if I wasn't trying to be healthy myself?

Having never considered the role of nutrition over and above avoiding deficiency, I naively assumed it was a simple case of 'eat less and move more'. But how? At the time, the advice to 'cut carbs' was rife within popular culture and among my colleagues, and so I adopted a low-carb diet in an attempt to lose body fat and feel healthier. I was eating a lot of chicken, fish and salads. I counted every calorie and threw myself into exercise. It worked. I lost a lot of weight and bought myself a new wardrobe. I felt pretty pleased with my efforts and new-found athleticism. From being the girl who would avoid sports at school at all costs, I was now running half marathons for the fun of it!

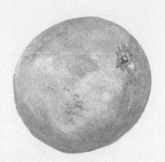

I felt that I was at my optimal health; surely this would set a benchmark for the rest of my life? It was at this point that I decided to do a health check blood test. This is a laboratory examination used to check for a variety of things, including the functioning of several organs, and gives an overall view of health. As a way of looking at the risk of heart disease, cholesterol and other proteins in the blood that carry fats (LDL, HDL and triglycerides) are also measured. This is known as a lipid panel.

I was shocked to discover that despite reducing my body fat, my blood test showed that my lipids were raised. Lipids are fat-like substances found in your blood and tissues; the main one is cholesterol. Your body needs small amounts of lipids to work normally and make hormones, but excess amounts can cause fatty deposits on the artery walls, increasing the risk of heart disease.

I have a history of heart disease in my family. My grandfather died from a heart attack while playing tennis. My father died of a heart attack at the age of only 59. Neither man was obese. I saw my results and I was dismayed. I chalked it up to my genetic destiny: if that was the hand I had been dealt, then there was nothing more I could do about it.

After my husband had his dramatic improvement with marathon running, I learned more about how to reduce inflammation and oxidative stress through diet. I wondered if there was a way to reverse my fate and take control of my own heart disease risk. I decided to go completely plant based and monitor what this did to my blood results.

I didn't tell anyone at first, not even my husband. What if I found it too hard or I lost my way? But I did it. And whether it was because I had done so much research already, or just because it felt so good, it was not half as challenging as I thought it would be. However, I recognised that my mini-experiment was not enough evidence by itself. When I turned to the literature, I found that others had achieved similar results time and again when they adopted a wholefoods plant-based diet. Why? Well, in a wholefoods, plant-based diet there is very little saturated fat, no dietary cholesterol, and abundant fibre, phytonutrients and antioxidants – which all work together to help blood vessels become more supple and responsive.

I was delighted and wanted to keep building on my personal evidence that a plant-based diet could get quick and effective results. I had read about it in studies, witnessed its benefits for my husband's health and fitness and now had seen how it had helped me. These markers for chronic disease tend to increase over time rather than decrease but now, ten years and two children later and with less time for exercise, when I have retested my lipid panel it is still normal, and I continue to be healthier than I was before.

It took that final personal experience to tip me into action. I realised I had some control over my genetic destiny. That although my genes loaded the gun, they did not pull the trigger. I felt I had a second chance at a long and healthy life.

THE FIRST PATIENT

After months of research and reviewing decades of international data, I decided to take the plunge and share some of the knowledge I had built up.

Richard and I had talked to family and friends about our plant-based discoveries. Many of them had acted as test cases for me and had reaped the benefits: dental abscesses had cleared up, diverticular disease pains had melted away, arthritis aches had disappeared.

But, was I brave enough to suggest plant-based eating in my consulting room?

One day, a middle-aged South African man walked into the office. He looked completely distraught. He sat down, turned to me and said, 'I've been sent home from work and I've been told not to come back.'

I had no idea where he was going to go with this, so asked cautiously, 'What happened?'

He explained that he was a driver at the airport and he had had a random spot medical. His blood pressure was sky high and he was told he couldn't drive, that his employers would inform the DVLA

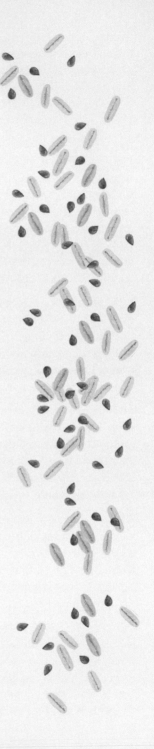

and his licence would be revoked. He would need a full medical and a normal blood pressure reading before he was allowed to return to work.

What is blood pressure? It is a reading expressed by two numbers, with one number on top (systolic) and the other number on the bottom (diastolic), like a fraction. The top number refers to the amount of pressure on your arteries during the contraction of your heart muscle and the bottom number refers to the pressure on the arteries between beats. High numbers indicate your heart is working too hard to pump blood to the rest of your body. A normal reading is around 120/80mmHg. This man's reading was 200/100mmHg, so we were talking about the need for major intervention otherwise he was at risk of having a stroke. In time, this extra pressure leads to an increased risk of kidney disease, dementia and erectile dysfunction as well as heart disease.

I described to him how we were likely to need to use three separate tablets, and gradually increase the doses in the hope that these medications may get the problem under control. He was devastated that there was no faster fix and didn't want to use medication. When I asked what he would like to do, all he said was that he wanted to go back to work.

'Would you like me to tell you about plant-based nutrition?' I began.

'What's that?' he asked.

He was not obese and there was no issue with his weight, but he ate a lot of red meat. I explained more and advised him on food groups to enjoy and gave him a few recipe ideas. I asked him to try a wholefoods plant-based diet and a couple of tablespoons of flax seeds crushed into a powder each day because I had read that it could be as effective in some people at reducing blood pressure as medication.

'OK, I'll give this plant thing a try,' he said. 'I'll do anything to be able to go back to work.'

He agreed to come back in a week so I could check his results. If there was no improvement, we would have to consider medication. He came back to see me the following week and I took his blood pressure. I couldn't believe what I was seeing. At 120/80mmHg, it was completely normal. Despite all I had learned, I was stunned at the level of improvement, and I brought him back to the surgery three times to check it wasn't a one-off. Sure enough, it continued to stay completely normal. I was able to do his medical for him and he went back to the job he loved.

From then on, if patients are interested in hearing more about plant-based nutrition, I share the benefits with them alongside prescribing normal medications, and I continue to see complete transformations. I look after thousands of patients and I want nothing more than to help people to get to grips with their health. In countless cases, eating a wholefood plant-based diet has helped them to do this. From young women suffering from hormone issues such as fibroids and endometriosis to older men with issues such as chronic pain, kidney disease, diabetes and depression, I continue to witness the transformative effects of a wholefoods plant-based lifestyle.

One lifestyle change is never going to be a panacea but what has been fascinating to observe is the unexpected 'side effects' of a plant-focused diet. One woman did it to improve her kidney function and her Crohn's disease improved and another man aimed to improve his arthritis pains and his prostate cancer regressed. These are the kind of side effects I would much prefer to live with!

HOW TO USE THIS BOOK

This book is designed to tell you everything you need to know about wholefoods plant-based living to help you feel empowered to make positive changes with a simple, actionable plan. I believe the information within these pages is life-changing and can help guide you to a life with more happiness, vitality and meaning.

In the first section, I will talk about what a plant-based diet really means, its incredible benefits for health and well-being, and why it is so important now more than ever.

Then I will show you how specific diseases respond to a healthy plant-based diet. You'll get an understanding of its power, and hopefully feel inspired to give it a try. I'll talk about how to get started with plant-based nutrition, budgeting, swaps and ensuring you and your family get the right nutrition that you need for your stage of life. In order to inspire you, I have created some recipes to provide some ideas to kick-start your journey.

Well-being is of course about so much more than what we put on our plates. But food is usually the first place that we begin. It can open our eyes to looking after ourselves in other ways. Loving more, stressing less, gratitude, movement, sleep and purpose are all foundational to health too. So, this book will also offer hints and tips throughout that will encourage you towards a complete view of health – the idea that it's not just what we eat, but how we live every day that can improve our health long term.

The purpose of this book is simple: to show you how you can make changes to your diet and lifestyle so you can heal from the inside out for optimum health. I want to share the tools and knowledge that I have learned.

I want to say a huge thank you for buying this book. Buying any book about changing your life in some way is a leap of faith. I hope this first leap will inspire you to many more strides forward in health, happiness and feeling more alive.

This is your book. So you must take from it what is most important to you. For some, that will be diving into the science and references. For others, it will be taking a feeling of what can fit into their life from within these pages, and applying it. Even taking one nugget of information and sharing it with your loved ones, or easing it into your life every day, will shift something in you. And those you love will notice it too.

What is it that you want? Think about this question before you read the book. You might find after reading it that there is something here that will get you closer to the answer to this question.

I love hearing inspiring stories from my patients. When they share their stories with me, it reminds me how much they have taught me over the years with their resilience, their spirit and their determination to feel better. My patients have found that simple swaps and shifts in daily habits, confidence and perspective have created massive changes for them. In many cases, these changes have given them their lives back.

This is what I hope for you: that you can really understand the power that you have. You are in control. If this book inspires you, please share your story with me. I would love to hear from you.

You can learn more about the work I do at www.plantpowerdoctor. com, where you will find my podcasts, blog posts, social media channels, free email subscription, and online courses and resources to help you continue in your journey. Wherever that leads you.

THE PLANT-POWER LIFESTYLE

'There comes a point where we need to stop just pulling people out of the river. We need to go upstream and find out why they're falling in.'

Archbishop Desmond Tutu

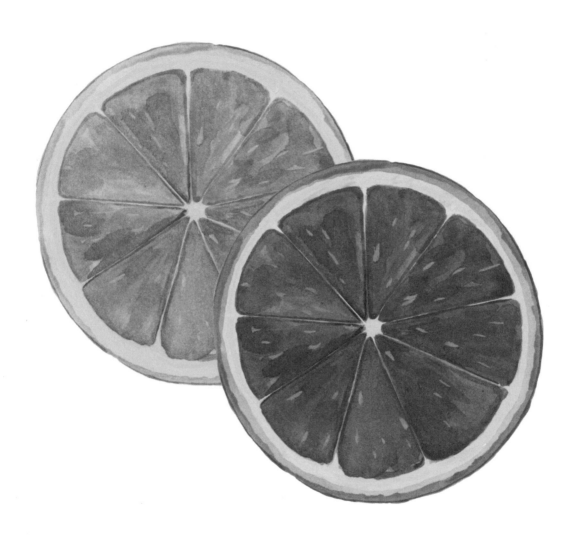

WHAT IS A WHOLEFOODS PLANT-BASED DIET?

Wholefoods are foods that are in their natural form, not heavily processed and with unrefined (or minimally refined) ingredients. Plant-based refers to food that comes from plants, which includes fruits, vegetables, beans and legumes, wholegrains, and nuts and seeds. A wholefoods plant-based diet does not include foods from animal sources, such as meat, dairy and eggs. From now on, if I am talking about a wholefoods, plant-based lifestyle, I will refer to it as a WFPB diet.

When you are eating 'plant-based' you simply commit to adding more of these plant-based foods to each meal for a 'plant-forward' or 'plant-heavy' approach. These plants and wholefoods play a starring role and the more and higher proportion of plants and wholefoods you eat, the more benefits you will see. I think of it as a natural and healthy style of eating.

My hope is that by sharing the plant-power principles, you can choose to follow them and notice how you feel. You may well notice health benefits you had not expected. I encourage you, as I do my patients, to jump in with both feet and see where it leads!

The beauty of a WFPB approach is that there is so much in the way of healthy, nourishing and delicious food choices once you know the basics, and unlike a 'diet' there is no need to restrict calories or worry about portion sizes. Many people find they can achieve an instinctive and healthy relationship with food by choosing WFPB eating, and eating when they're hungry. You won't feel deprived or go hungry, and the high-fibre content means your digestive system will be as happy as your taste buds.

Remember: this book is not about feeling restricted. With that principle in mind, I do not want you to feel you have failed if you don't follow a WFPB diet to the letter. There is a certain type of all-or-nothing thinking many people are prone to, where if we make a mistake, we are tempted to pack it all in. Don't fall victim to this; every step in the right direction is a step to feel proud of. The goal is to feel good in your body and mind.

You can feel confident that the advice is healthy and evidence based. The suggestions I make are based on decades of international research, and the aim is to optimise health, suit any budget – and to consider what is sustainable for our planet.

I am confident that, in sharing this with you, I am following a large body of data and peer-reviewed guidelines to bring you information that your doctor, friend or relative may not have seen, and that could have the power to change your health.

I encourage you to share your results with your own doctor too. They may well find themselves surprised and encouraged by the changes they see in you, and it could even inspire them to talk more about the benefits of nutrition and lifestyle with other patients. There's a reason I am one of the happiest doctors I know: nothing brings more job satisfaction for a doctor than seeing your patients take control of their lives and their health. Wanting to help people is the reason most doctors go into medicine. My hope is that this book will do exactly that for you, without the need for a prescription pad.

In this book, I will guide you through an exploration of why our bodies respond well to plant-based eating. We will discover examples of some of the most common health issues that face us today, and how they can be improved using plant-based nutrition.

Below is an overview of the principles we will take away and that I hope will help you make a start in your plant-power life:

- Everyone needs to cut down their meat consumption. We eat too much protein and not enough fibre. For adults, the Department of Health recommends no more than 70g red and processed meat a day – the average pork sausage weighs 75g so is already over the daily maximum allowance. Cutting out meat could help with a host of health conditions.

● Dairy is a source of calcium and nutrients but it is not necessary to consume it as part of a balanced diet. The Canadian Dietary Guidelines for 2019 exclude dairy. Some dairy products, such as cheese, are naturally high in fat and consumption of dairy products has also been linked to some health conditions, such as eczema and prostate cancer.

● If you are turning to this book because you have a chronic illness and are seeking health improvements, this does not replace the medical advice of your own doctor. A well-planned WFPB approach is known to be a really healthy choice, and every step in the direction of a plant-forward, plant-strong approach will provide benefits; you will discover what works best for you.

● If you are very ill and/or can't cook, and want to buy ready-made plant-based options, then look at the labels. You will see the nutritional information per serving on the back or the side of the packaging. It is important to remember that portion sizes on the label may not reflect the amount you are eating. Where colour coded with traffic light labels, you can see at a glance whether they are high, medium or low in fat, saturated fat, sugars and salt. For a healthier choice, pick products with more greens and ambers. Try to avoid foods with any red labels. Pre-packaged foods will also have a list of ingredients and this can help you work out how healthy the product is. Ingredients are listed in order of weight, so the main ingredients will come first. As a rule of thumb, the fewer ingredients the better. Once you are feeling more energised, wholefoods cooked from scratch are fantastic and hopefully you'll be inspired to cook some of the recipes in this book, as well as the many simple WFPB recipes available in other cookbooks and online.

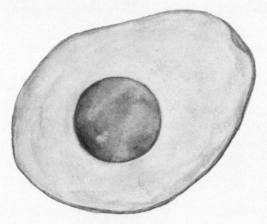

A WHOLE HEALTH VIEW

Five blindfolded doctors are asked to describe an elephant standing right in front of them. They get really close and start to touch the body part nearest to them. 'A tree!' exclaims the doctor with her hands on the elephant's trunk. 'A rope!' says the doctor who has grabbed the elephant's tail. 'A fan!', 'A wall!', 'A pillar' they shout. Each is convinced of their assessment, and that they alone are correct.

In medicine, we don't have five blindfolded doctors, we have thousands of researchers performing studies looking at only one aspect of the elephant, each through a different pair of glasses. That is a good thing because in science we need specific answers to specific questions. But it is only when we piece all the perspectives together that we begin to see the true shape of the elephant in the room.

In health and wellness, that elephant in the room is the fact that our health as a population is affected by the food we eat. In 2017, 11 million deaths worldwide were caused by what we eat, and what we don't. High intake of salt, low intake of wholegrains and low intake of fruits were the leading dietary risk factors for deaths globally. In environmental science, the elephant in the room is that the ecosystems on which we and all other species depend are deteriorating more rapidly than ever.

The good news is that in finding solutions that can improve our health and our resilience to disease, we can also improve the biodiversity of the planet. With a 'wholeistic' view we can see many levels of benefits can be achieved by eating more plants. In 2019, the EAT Lancet Commission was created to think about the two elephants in the room. A group of 37 nutritional scientists from across the globe were tasked with creating food guidelines to include the 2.1 billion people who are overweight and obese and the 821 million people who go hungry. They had to look at the reality of what we actually have right now in terms of global ecology, agricultural systems and increasing overpopulation, and ask 'what could we do that would avoid the complete collapse of our planet's ability to support our species?' The answer – a predominantly plant-based diet. To reach their recommendations, the UK and Ireland would have to make a dramatic reduction in meat and dairy consumption.

Perhaps you have turned to this book because you are battling with some big health issues. Worrying about the planet might feel like too much of a burden in addition to this. That's OK. Focus on improving your health, safe in the knowledge that by eating a wholefoods plant-based diet, you are tackling both elephants in the room.

WHAT IS A 'HEALTHY' DIET?

There is more than one way to eat healthily, just as there is more than one way to eat unhealthily. There has always been a lot of confusion around diets and nutrition. The media, food companies, government and even health professionals give differing advice about our diet and health. We see it on TV and in the newspapers every week: one week coffee causes cancer and the next week it prevents it. Low fat, low carbohydrate, keto, paleo – which diet is the healthy choice when the headlines change so often? I have always found this the most frustrating part of helping patients with lifestyle change – when headlines and fads grab their attention, and ultimately make them feel miserable and think they have failed when they don't get that 'bikini body' or lose those extra pounds.

How do we cut through the noise? I like to look at the findings of large, independent bodies of research to help with this. The 'True Health Initiative' brought together over 100 experts from more than 30 countries to create a consensus. This is one example of a reliable source to help us understand how lifestyle can reduce the impact of chronic disease.

What did they agree on? Along with regular exercise and adequate sleep, they agreed that **a diet rich in vegetables, fruits, nuts, seeds, wholegrains and water remains the cornerstone of good health.** I read this research and felt relieved. Someone was willing to take a step back from the fads and the nutritional tribes and share a wholistic approach to food.

You must decide what feels right for you. Most importantly, you – and only you – can decide what it is you feel you can include and maintain as a habit in your life, rather than a 'quick-fix'. But by increasing your intake of plant-based wholefoods, the evidence shows you can only do good for your health long term.

WHAT'S HEALTHY FOR YOU?

Many experts have contributed their wisdom and experience to this book, including dieticians, nutritionists and fellow medical doctors, and I am very grateful to them. I could not have compiled this book alone. Rest assured you can trust the information here, which is based on years of research – this is no fad diet. What I do want to make clear though, is this book isn't the same as you visiting me for a consultation. I don't know your specific health requirements and history. Use this book as an introduction to understand why what you eat is important to how you feel. For a bespoke plan, please continue the conversation with a dietician, nutritionist or doctor and find a way of eating and living that suits your specific health needs.

IS A WFPB DIET THE SAME AS VEGANISM?

WFPB lifestyles and veganism share many similarities, but there is a difference. Veganism seeks to exclude, as far as is practical, all animal products from all aspects of living. Vegan clothing, cleaning products and make-up also avoid the use of animals in testing or for ingredients. As a vegan, you will benefit from eating more fruits and vegetables and removing animal products, but a vegan diet could also include processed food, such as crisps, sodas and sweets.

As veganism booms in popularity, so does the availability of vegan meat substitutes and ready prepared foods. From 'no-chicken' chicken nuggets to vegan desserts, there are now many options, but they may not always be better for your health. Just because these products are labelled plant-based doesn't mean they won't contain too much sugar, salt or fat. When thinking about a healthy choice on your own plate, it helps to compare it to what you would otherwise have eaten. A mushroom sausage will be healthier than a pork sausage – more plant nutrients, less fat and salt. But when you compare a meat replacement burger with a vegan cheese and bean burger, the benefits are not so clear-cut – some vegan substitutes are high in salt and/or sugar and may contain artificial ingredients, preservatives and processed oils.

A WFPB diet emphasises fresh, nutritious and minimally processed foods. The closer your food choices are to their natural state, the better.

WHY IS A WFPB DIET HEALTHY?

An apple a day keeps the doctor away. That's what Granny used to say. Everyone knows fruit and vegetables are important and crucial to good health. But why exactly is that?

Fruit and vegetables are full of antioxidants, vitamins, minerals, fibre and phytochemicals, which are many thousands of compounds working in synergy to create wellness, and many of which we are yet to discover. Fruit and vegetables, along with wholegrains and beans, are our only sources of dietary fibre, which plays an important role in our health (more on fibre later).

What are phytochemicals? These are naturally occurring chemicals produced by plants, and they are responsible for the colour, flavour and smell of the plant – such as the rich colours of blueberries and tomatoes, the incredible bite of a chilli pepper and the slightly bitter taste of broccoli. Phytochemicals function to protect plants against invasion, the sun's rays, disease and infection but they can also do us a lot of good too.

As one example, carotenoids are a class of phytochemicals with more than 600 naturally occurring pigments. Carotenoids are found in the most richly coloured yellow, orange and red fruits and vegetables like pumpkin, tomatoes, bell peppers, mangos, tangerines, carrots, squash and watermelons. Alpha-carotene, beta-carotene, lutein, lycopene and zeaxathin are the most common carotenoids in foods. In our bodies, they act as antioxidants and have anti-inflammatory and immune-system benefits. Beta-carotene found in carrots and other fruits and veggies can be converted to vitamin A and is important for maintaining eye health.

Tens of thousands of phytochemicals have been discovered but there are many we do not know about yet and we are only just beginning to understand what they can do for human health and their far-reaching impact. Most plant foods contain many – carrots, for example, have over 100 – and they all do different things and complement each other.

EATING THE RAINBOW

Nature offers us a vibrant and exciting colour palette and 'eating the rainbow' is the best way to ensure that you are eating a wide variety of phytochemicals.

Evidence shows that taking phytochemicals in supplement form may not provide the same benefits. Larger concentrations of phytochemicals are found in all the edible parts of plants, especially in the skin and peel. For example, a raw unpeeled apple contains up to 332 per cent more vitamin K, 142 per cent more vitamin A, 115 per cent more vitamin C, 20 per cent more calcium and up to 19 per cent more potassium than a peeled apple. My patients often talk about how vibrant their plates have become by moving away from beige foods to eating a variety of rainbow-coloured fruit and vegetables.

I've listed a host of colourful fruit and veg to help get you started and inspire your next food shop on page 148.

THE WFPB DIET AND CHRONIC DISEASE

Let's look in more detail at how plants can help with a range of common health issues and chronic diseases.

If the WFPB was a pill, just how healthy would it be?

Let's pretend that all its effects could be achieved through a pill. The pharmaceutical company that has developed and patented this drug holds a big press conference and unveils all the therapeutic benefits of their new medication.

It can:

- Reduce inflammation.
- Help slow the ageing process.
- Improve the chances of reaching a healthy weight through diet.

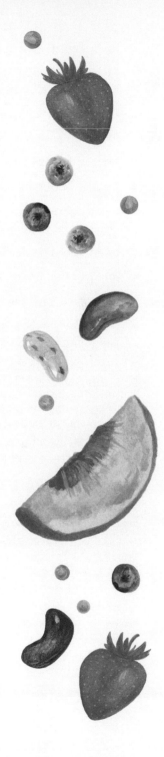

- Reduce the risk of developing heart disease.

- Reduce the risk of developing the vast majority of cancers and help us recover from cancer treatment.

- Prevent us developing Type 2 diabetes and help us reverse it.

- Improve our mental health.

- Maintain a healthy gut, eliminate diverticular disease and IBS.

- Balance our hormones and keep the thyroid healthy.

- Reduce period pains, increase our fertility and reduce menopausal symptoms.

- Improve erectile function and increase sperm count.

- Improve skin health, acne and eczema.

- Strengthen immunity.

- Help alleviate the symptoms of rheumatoid arthritis, lupus and multiple sclerosis.

Imagine all of those health benefits in just one drug – it would be worth millions!

I'm sorry there is no magic pill. But the good news is that anyone can follow a WFPB diet and get these kinds of improvements. Let's look in more detail to understand why what you put on the end of your fork matters so much.

INFLAMMATION

When doctors talk about inflammation and eating anti-inflammatory foods, what are they talking about? Think of it in terms of your skin. Have you ever been stung by a bee or got a splinter stuck in your finger? Did you notice how it becomes red, warm, inflamed and painful? This is the body's inflammatory response at work – one of the most brilliantly designed systems we know. It leaps into action when danger is detected to combat bacteria and viruses that might have entered the body and takes emergency measures to remove them. You will notice that when you have finally plucked the splinter or sting out, the inflammation quietens down and the body heals the small wound.

We live in a world where we are overloaded by long-term stressors like anxiety, lack of sleep, poor diet and environmental toxins. As a result, the inflammatory response goes into overdrive and becomes a long-lasting 'habit', even when there is no injury or disease. This can lead to chronic low-level inflammation throughout your body.

When I talk about something being 'chronic', it refers to a condition that is persistent or long-lasting and is often used to describe any illness that lasts for more than three months. Chronic inflammation is inflammation that sticks around for longer than it's needed. This means that chronic inflammation initiated by lifestyle factors can then become a starting point for disease. It plays a central role in almost every major disease, including cancer, heart disease, diabetes, Alzheimer's disease and even depression.

WHAT CAUSES INFLAMMATION?

- Trans fats
- Animal fats
- High-fat diet
- Stress
- Smoking
- Sleep deprivation
- Obesity and weight gain
- Excessive calorie intake
- Sugar-sweetened drinks
- High-salt diet
- Low fibre consumption
- Excessive alcohol

One of the main areas of the body affected by this chronic low-level inflammation is your 100,000 kilometres of blood vessels (if laid out this would be two and a half times around the Earth!).

The well-being of your circulatory system is crucial for many aspects of your health. If the immune response triggers white blood cells but they have nothing to do and nowhere to go, this can cause lasting damage to tissues and organs. For example, inflammatory cells that spend too long in blood vessels promote the build-up of dangerous plaque. As the plaque continues to build, this can cause your arteries to thicken, increasing the risk of heart disease and stroke.

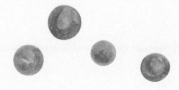

HOW CAN WE COMBAT INFLAMMATION?

How we respond to inflammation varies from person to person because our genetics, our microbiome – the variety of bugs that live within us, especially in our gut – and our immune system are as unique as our fingerprints. But there are various ways you can adopt healthy lifestyle habits to have a positive effect on inflammation. These include regular exercise, keeping our BMI at a healthy level and sleeping well. What about the foods we eat? By loading up on anti-inflammatory foods, such as colourful fruit and vegetables, we are giving our bodies a powerful weapon to fight inflammation. If free radicals in the body are like small fires, imagine the antioxidants in fruit and vegetables as tiny fire engines putting them out.

There are plenty of foods that have been found to reduce inflammation, but many of them have been studied in the lab rather than in people: foods such as turmeric, blueberries, ginger, tea, dark chocolate and various vegetables to name a few!

What do studies of real people show? Two epidemiologists surveyed 1,943 studies and published a Dietary Inflammatory Index with 45 food elements. They created it as a research tool for evaluating diets, and showed that fruit and vegetables, fibre, turmeric, ginger, garlic and omega-3 fatty acids were consistently anti-inflammatory. In contrast, excess calories, protein, iron, trans fats and saturated fats had the opposite effect.

TOP TIPS TO CURB INFLAMMATION

- Eating plenty of fruit and vegetables.
- Enjoying herbs and spices.
- Physical activity.
- Going barefoot outside.
- Not eating too much.
- Drinking plenty of water.
- Eating a high-fibre diet.
- Prioritising good sleep.

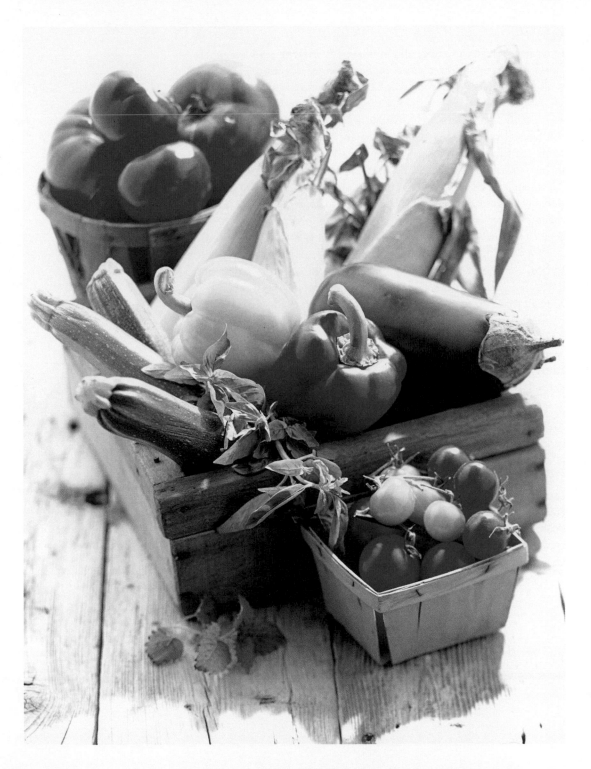

WHY IS A WFPB DIET HEALTHY?

OXIDATIVE STRESS

Oxidative stress can affect all kinds of body systems and is a main cause of inflammation, cardiovascular disease, infection, cancer and even ageing. The process of oxidation happens as our bodies metabolise (or process) the oxygen we breathe, and our cells produce energy from it. These natural body processes cause our mitochondria – the tiny structures in our cells that act like batteries to power them – to release something called free radicals. So, in order to create energy, we cannot avoid also producing free radicals. These are reactive oxygen species that are produced by the body during metabolic processes. They are a bit like pinballs in a pinball machine because they are small and fast moving and as they move, they can cause damage to our cells and tissues. What they need in order to stop damaging us, is the donation of electrons. You see, free radicals are positively charged oxygen, and they need to pair with a negative charge (from electrons) to return balance to the body. We call these electrons antioxidants. In general, the body is able to maintain a balance between antioxidants and free radicals, but not always. An imbalance – where the number of free radicals produced overwhelms the repair process – can cause stress inside our cells and cause us to age prematurely.

Remember, oxidation happens when our cells use glucose to make energy, when the immune system is in action and when our body detoxifies pollutants, such as cigarette smoke. Other reasons for oxidative stress include things you may think of as being 'unhealthy': sitting too much, sleeping too little, lack of exercise, stress, eating refined foods and animal products. By eating a WFPB diet, you can think of the compounds in plant foods – or polphenols – as mini electron donators, and in a series of chemical reactions inside our cells, the electrons from plant foods are released and donated to us. So now, when you hear that blueberries are antioxidants, you'll know why.

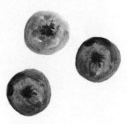

THE GREAT FIBRE PROVIDER

It is a sad reality that only 5 per cent of us eat as much fibre as we need, which can lead to all sorts of problems. In fact, most of us get almost half the recommended daily amount (18g when ideally we should be getting 30g). Why is fibre the forgotten dietary essential?

Dietary fibre is probably best known for keeping the digestion system moving and preventing constipation. This is because it is made from complex structures that cannot be broken down by the human digestive system, so fibre passes through it and helps waste flow. But just because we can't digest this fibre, it doesn't mean we can't use it. Having a diet with plenty of fibre offers many health benefits, including maintaining a healthy weight and lowering your risk of diabetes, heart disease and some kinds of cancers. In the 1960s, a surgeon called Denis Burkitt (who discovered Burkitt's lymphoma) found that Ugandans who ate high-fibre vegetable diets avoided many common diseases of Europeans and Americans, such as diabetes, irritable bowel syndrome (IBS), constipation, diverticular disease, colon cancer and heart disease. After looking at many factors, he concluded that a high amount of fibre is necessary for maintaining good health.

Since then, huge amounts of further research have been done in this area showing the benefits of high-fibre foods. Many of these previously unknown benefits are down to the fact that fibre is crucial food for our beneficial gut microbiota. These gut bugs are our internal ecosystem of millions of microbes, including bacteria, viruses and fungi, that live in our intestines and outnumber our own body's cells by 10 to 1. These bacteria are crucial and play a key role in digesting the food we eat, as well as absorbing and synthesising nutrients. Their influence extends well beyond the gut, impacting our metabolism, mood, body weight and immune function too. So, when we eat fibre we are not only feeding ourselves, but also keeping our gut bugs alive and well nourished. Fibre only comes from plant foods – think fruits, vegetables, wholegrains and beans. I will talk more about the unique benefits of fibre on pages 63–4, 77 and 117–18.

LONGEVITY – WHO LIVES TO 100?

We all want to live long and healthy lives but how much is dictated by our lifestyle and how much by our genes? There are some clues in a handful of magical places where the number of people living to 100 is up to ten times higher than the rest of the world. In these places – Okinawa (Japan); Sardinia (Italy); Nicoya (Costa Rica); Icaria (Greece) and among the Seventh-day Adventists in Loma Linda (California) – the people tend to be very healthy and are active into their eighties and nineties but they have much lower rates of chronic disease, so they not only live longer but live better. These areas were named the 'Blue Zones' by National Geographic researcher Dan Buettner.

One major factor explaining this phenomenon is that these people share an important eating habit in common – a 95 per cent plant-based diet. The average menu in each place is very different, but there are parallels among the core ingredients. The foods they have in common are nuts and seeds, healthy wholegrains and lots of vegetables alongside a cup of beans, legumes or pulses per day. So, despite the enormous variety in the culture and style of their diets, they see similar results.

The Blue Zones also share important lifestyle similarities, such as making movement throughout the day a natural way of life, having purpose, being part of faith-based communities and sharing strong family links, as well as including stress-relieving habits in their day (more on all of this later).

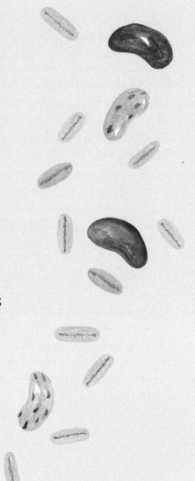

WHY DOES OXIDATION AGE US?

One way we age is through the effect of oxidation on our DNA. The DNA building blocks inside the nucleus of every cell in our bodies twist into neat and compact chromosomes, which house all our genetic material. Telomeres are the caps on the end of our chromosomes, which stop them from sticking together when cells divide. You can think of telomeres as protectors, like caps on the ends of our shoelaces to stop them from fraying. The average cell divides about 60 times before it dies, and each time this happens, the telomere caps on the end of the chromosomes get shorter and shorter. When they get too short, the cell dies. Oxidative stress can shorten the length of our telomeres.

Studies have shown that people with long telomeres live longer and healthier lives than people with short telomeres. Interestingly, Elizabeth Blackburn, a Nobel Prize-winning scientist, did a study which found that just three months of eating a plant-based diet significantly boosted telomerase activity. Telomerase is an enzyme that helps maintain the length of these protective telomeres. In a follow-up study, telomere length was noted to have actually increased in the plant-based diet group. While the group eating plant foods also exercised and lost weight, other studies have shown that even more vigorous exercise and similar amounts of weight loss have not affected telomere length in this way. What does this mean? That eating more plants can make us younger, at least on the level of our cells.

Let's look at oxidative stress in terms our blood vessels. They have an inner layer of cells called the endothelial lining that does an incredible job; it produces something called nitric oxide, one of the most important molecules for blood vessel health. Nitric oxide massively reduces oxidative stress and is a powerful vasodilator, meaning that it helps your blood vessels stay lovely and supple. It has an anti-inflammatory effect by preventing damage to your blood vessel lining, and an anti-clotting effect by stopping blood platelets from sticking to blood vessel walls. This reduces your risk of high blood pressure, which then lessens your risk of heart disease long term. Nitric oxide also has a role in making insulin more effective by grabbing glucose from the bloodstream and putting it into the cell more easily. Therefore, good nitric oxide levels reduce both heart disease and diabetes risk.

How does a plant-based diet help the blood vessels get enough nitric oxide? Vegetables, particularly leafy greens, contain nitrate, which can be converted in the body to nitrites and then to nitric oxide. The polyphenols in plants can also increase nitric oxide production in the body. This means that plants can provide what the body needs to reduce oxidative stress.

WHAT ELSE CAN AFFECT AGEING?

Another process in the body that can age us is the activation of an ageing enzyme called TOR, which stands for 'target of rapamycin'. Rapamycin is a drug that suppresses the immune system and is given to transplant patients to prevent the body from rejecting new organs. It also inhibits the ageing enzyme TOR. When this enzyme TOR is activated, cells grow and divide, but when it's turned down, cells go into conservation mode and clean up and recycle old proteins. TOR-driven ageing is a bit like an engine on a car going at full speed without brakes. When we are young, the engine is supposed to run like this, but as we age the car must slow down, and problems arise if the car continues at 100mph. TOR is absolutely necessary when we are young, but is implicated in cancer, heart disease, diabetes, Alzheimer's and other diseases as we get older.

Changing our diet may be the best way to slow down TOR. Caloric restriction can inhibit TOR, but this is difficult to sustain long term. Is there an easier way? Increasing your intake of plant foods can help. Eating less animal protein has been shown to dampen down TOR activity, mimicking the effects of energy restriction, but without the side effects. Amazingly, fruits and vegetables have phytochemicals that function as natural TOR inhibitors too. The cancer-protective effect of WFPB diets is thought to be in part due to this anti-ageing effect.

Of course, it's important to remember that ageing is complex. Aside from the factors we have covered, oxidative stress, telomere shortening and TOR pathway signalling, there are lots of other elements involved – like genetics, stress and our environment. But the food you eat can make a big difference and could be the most important factor you have the power to change every day. Medical advances, cosmetic procedures and scientific discoveries are all helping us to live longer, but cellular science and the Blue Zones research show us that plants could be the simplest way to live longer and healthier lives.

EAT MORE AND WEIGH LESS

Let's talk about weight. This is a hugely complex issue and one that has played a big part in my health journey. I used to be much bigger than I am now. I was happy, but heavier than is healthy for longevity and for a long time I struggled to see results.

For lots of people, weight is not just a simple equation of food in and energy out, but determined by a whole host of external and personal factors, from our food environment, what shops we have access to, our upbringing, whether or not we smoke, how much alcohol we consume, if we do shift work and how stressed we are to our genetics, medications, sleep patterns and so much more. Even if you do follow a pattern of trying to burn more calories than you eat, this can be hard to maintain.

We live in a world where more people die from complications relating to obesity than malnutrition. In a 2017 survey, it was found that 28.7 per cent of adults in the UK are obese and a further 35.6 per cent are overweight. This is the problem of this generation; the worldwide prevalence of obesity nearly tripled between 1975 and 2016. Diseases relating to obesity include diabetes, heart disease, some cancers, dementia, liver disease, polycystic ovarian syndrome and mental health problems.

Despite being overfed, many of us who are overweight are in fact undernourished. Why? Because a lot of the most inexpensive meals are also highly processed and energy-dense, packed with fat, refined grains and sugars. Unhealthier foods are often on special offer and are promoted as being very convenient. However, they don't always have the nutrients our bodies need. This is not our fault; our food environment is stacked against us.

Weight is a big problem for many of us. Being kind and understanding the causes is important. Very few of us 'want' to be unhealthily overweight. But many people, including doctors, still lack the right knowledge about nutrition and weight gain. We know that poor diet and inactivity are drivers of weight gain but there are many other factors at play.

Research tells us that on average, we make around 15 conscious food choices each day, but well over 200 unconscious ones. Supermarkets, town planners, billboard ad companies and government policy makers should all be involved in helping us to access healthy food choices that don't cost the earth. This is especially true in poorer areas where people may find it hard to seek out healthy foods let alone cook them. Society needs to make it easy to be healthy. But until then, what's the easiest way to help ourselves?

CALORIES

Plants are nutrient rich and low in calories. Calorie density refers to the amount of calories per pound of a given food. This can range from 100 calories per pound in non-starchy vegetables to 4,000 calories per pound in some kinds of oils. Foods that have lower calorie density often also have higher nutrient density. Eating these types of foods also helps us get back to a more instinctive way of eating, so we remain full. Some of the most nutrient-rich foods include leafy greens like kale, beans, garlic, and blueberries. A WFPB diet is one of the most nutrient-dense patterns of eating, and will likely contain more folate, vitamin C, beta-carotene (for making vitamin A), riboflavin, thiamine, magnesium and potassium and less saturated fat and cholesterol than a meat-and-dairy-heavy diet.

WFPB diets are also packed with fibre, which helps to fill us up, without adding empty calories. Studies have shown that hunger hormones are an important part of regulating our appetite, and that having the right amount of them means we are more likely to feel full. Vegan and vegetarian diets have been shown to help curb hunger by improving levels of three key hunger hormones that we make, boosting our satiety. Much data now also exists showing that people who eat a plant-based diet or those who do not eat meat tend to have lower BMIs than those who do eat animal products. This is important because we all want to make it easier to be in a healthy weight range, and for many people, a WFPB diet is a great way to achieve this while also feeling we have had as much as we wanted to eat.

Eating foods with a reduced caloric density combined with increased nutrient density and fibre is a wonderful way to lose weight. It greatly simplifies the sums of energy in versus energy out. This is another reason why WFPB approaches tend to limit oils too: there are a lot more calories per spoon of oil compared to the same amount of energy and nutrients from the wholefood. With a WFPB approach, we give our bodies nutrients and satiety, which means cravings are minimised, so we can maintain a healthy weight and BMI more simply, and thereby reduce our risk of developing a number of diseases.

NO MORE DIETING

We all know that traditional diets do not work. You simply lose weight and then put it back on again, leading to a pattern of yo-yo dieting. Many people who go on diets end up gaining weight. Deprivation when you 'go on a diet' can lead to changes in hormones, metabolism and cognitive functions that make it difficult to keep the weight off. It can also disrupt the stability of our gut microbiome and, not least, leave us feeling frustrated and unsatisfied.

The beauty of a WFPB approach is that it is an eating pattern of abundance with no need for calorie counting and restriction or even trying to carefully calibrate your different intakes of nutrients. A common issue I have noticed in my patients is that dieters often feel hungrier. Their attention is biased toward food and research shows that they may even find food tastier. So stop dieting and start eating more plants.

There are many studies that highlight the benefits of WFPB nutrition for weight loss. One of my favourites is the BROAD study, one of the first of its kind. For the study, scientists took 33 people, and a similar-sized control group, and allowed them to eat whatever amount of food they wanted as long as it fitted into the WFPB guidelines they set up, which included an emphasis on wholegrains, legumes, vegetables and fruit.

Starches like sweet potatoes, bread and pasta were encouraged to help with feeling full, but consumption of oils, such as olive oil and coconut oil, animal products, high-fat foods and highly processed foods was discouraged. Participants were also asked to cut back on sugar, salt and caffeinated drinks. The participants undertook lifestyle education and cooking classes and were given vitamin B12 supplements. They were all assessed at six months and then a year.

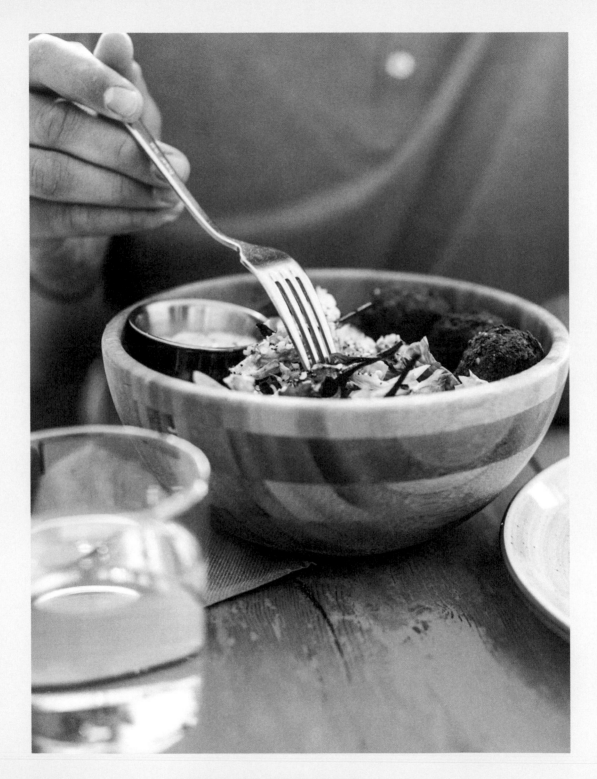

THE PLANT POWER DOCTOR

The subjects ended up losing and keeping off an average of 25 pounds – showing sustained and effective weight loss over a long time period, crucially without the need for caloric restriction or exercise. The trial took place in New Zealand in a region with high levels of poverty, obesity and Type 2 diabetes. Two out of the four patients with diabetes reduced their dosage or reliance on diabetes medications, including one who no longer required insulin. This research supports the idea that a WFPB diet is safe, sustainable and effective, and can be achieved cheaply if you have a limited budget.

Most people starting a WFPB lifestyle who are carrying extra weight will tend to lose weight naturally. If you are hoping to do so, these are my top tips:

Focus on healthy choices over losing weight: Studies show that having four healthy habits (eating five or more servings fruit/vegetables per day, limiting alcohol consumption, not smoking, and exercising over 12 times per month) reduces weight-based differences in early mortality. This means even if you are overweight, doing these four things will likely reduce your risk of dying younger. So instead of dieting, I suggest focusing on healthy choices – like enjoying vegetables – without worrying about reducing calories.

Fill up on veggies: Non-starchy veggies are the most nutrient dense and low calorie. Green leafy veggies like cabbage, spinach, kale and lettuce are particularly high in natural compounds called thylakoids that are thought to suppress appetite. Starchy veg help to fill us up, which is important for satiety, as well as giving us plenty of vitamins and minerals. They really add to the satisfaction of a meal.

Love legumes: The healthiest populations on the planet eat beans and pulses. They are a protein and fibre powerhouse and can even help reduce the sugar spike of other meals, and so are really helpful for people with diabetes too. Pulses are one aspect of a plant-based diet that can be new to people. They can cause bloating if you are not used to them. But be patient, trust me it's worth it! Start slowly, perhaps with split lentils, which are smaller. Rinsing pre-cooked pulses a couple of times or soaking and sprouting dry pulses can all be helpful if you have never tried a lentil before.

Happy wholegrains: Quinoa, barley, millet, oats, red rice, black rice and buckwheat are hugely beneficial in terms of protein, fibre and micronutrients. You might have been told to cut the carbs, but intact wholegrains are consistently valuable for health. Refined grains are stripped of a lot of the nutritional value, so it is worth limiting these whether you are aiming for weight loss or not.

Avoid liquid calories: Avoid drinking calories in sweetened drinks and opt for water or teas. Eating whole fruits will always be more nutritionally beneficial than drinking fruit juice. Vegetable juices like carrot and celery are a great way to boost phytonutrients, but be aware that fruit without the fibre is a lot of sugar to drink in one go.

Limit vegan junk food: Just because a product is labelled plant-based does not necessarily mean it is healthy. Many meat substitute foods are processed, dense in calories and lower in nutrients than whole foods. If you have these foods sometimes, take the time to enjoy them. Eating on the go or feeling guilty about less healthy foods is not helpful; food is supposed to be fun.

Limit alcohol: Most of us have a drink or two on special occasions, but studies show that alcohol use is a leading risk factor for increased risk of death from any cause, especially cancer, and the level that minimises loss of health is . . . zero. Yup. Even the polyphenols in red wine can't negate these findings. What a party pooper! Alcohol can be used as a way to relax after a hard day for some, but for others its use can so easily become unhealthy or even addictive. For all of us, alcohol is full of empty calories too, so if you are hoping to get to a healthy weight, it is an obvious thing to cut back on.

Avoid low-fat products: Many people associate low-fat foods with healthy foods but this is not always the case. Processed low-fat foods are often loaded with sugar and additives. Be aware that some wholefoods like nuts and avocados are high in calories but these can still be eaten in moderation as part of a balanced WFPB diet if you are trying to lose weight.

There are many delicious meals you can make that are healthy, easy and that follow a WFPB lifestyle, and can be enjoyed by the whole family. Later on in the book, I share some of my favourite recipes. No calorie counting involved!

HEART HEALTH

As a little girl, I loved nothing more than a hug from my 'Teddy Bear' Grandad. I called him that because of his comforting round belly, and his soft rumbling laugh that made me feel safe and loved. But as comforted as he made me feel, my cuddly grandad was not going to be able to keep himself from dying younger than he should. He died at 60 years old because of a mixture of heart disease and cancer, the Western world's two biggest killers. I often imagine the pride he would have felt had he been given the chance to meet my sons and give them his big grandad hugs too.

My dad's father also died as a result of a sudden heart attack, leaving my dad and grandmother devastated, and leaving this world well before his time. An active and slim man, no one expected that his heart arteries would be blocked, or that he would be here one day and gone the next.

Tragically, my dad was to suffer the same fate a few years later. He died suddenly of a heart attack at just 59 years of age. He never got the chance to meet his grandsons or be a part of their lives. There are many more stories like this, of loved ones lost, both from my own life and in the lives of my patients. We all must die and some of us will die before our time, despite having a healthy lifestyle. But heart disease in our fifties, sixties and seventies is not inevitable. Simply put, there is another way to eat and live.

HEART DISEASE

Do you know anyone with impotence, high blood pressure or heart disease? Chances are, you do. According to the British Heart Foundation (BHF), someone is hospitalised with a heart attack in the UK every three minutes. It is the UK's leading cause of death. So it is worth knowing about ways in which our risk of this fatal disease can be improved or even reversed using lifestyle interventions. The average heart pumps 60–80 beats per minute for our whole lives and when it stops, so do we. It pays to look after our hearts.

What is heart disease? Cardiovascular means heart and blood vessels. Heart disease is a general term for diseases of the blood vessels. This includes the vessels of the heart, which can be narrowed in angina, causing chest pain, or completely blocked in the case of a heart attack. A blockage of vessels in the brain can cause a stroke and narrowing of the vessels can cause dementia. Narrowing in the peripheral blood vessels can cause impotence if this happens in the penis, or peripheral vascular disease if this happens in the legs, causing pain when walking, ulcers, or even gangrene. Any vessel anywhere in the body can begin to stiffen, narrow and block, which is really the underlying problem in heart disease.

The bad news first. A study showed that even one high-fat milkshake has the power to change the shape of your blood cells and of the fat particles circulating in your bloodstream, leading to more oxidised low-density lipoproteins (LDL). These newly 'spiky' cells are a major carrier of circulating cholesterol and can potentially damage the thin layer of cells that line blood vessels, called the endothelial lining. Although the cells recover in a few hours, imagine having this every meal, every day, for the rest of your life. These changes become pathological and unstable plaques form in your blood vessels. These fatty deposits cling to artery walls and can clog them, making it more likely that a blood clot will form. Accumulated over a lifetime, this leads to an increased risk of clotting and stroke, heart attack and untimely death.

The good news: we can change our chances of getting heart disease through lifestyle. A WFPB diet will:

Support healthy cholesterol levels and cut out saturated fat

Diets high in saturated fats raise cholesterol levels. Foods high in saturated fat sometimes trigger the body into producing more cholesterol. It is thought that one of the reasons a WFPB diet can be so effective for supporting heart health is because plants do not contain any dietary cholesterol and almost never contain saturated fat. The plant 'cholesterol' that they do contain (phytosterols) can block cholesterol from being absorbed by the body. They are also rich in fibre, which helps to lower cholesterol. Soluble fibre slows the absorption of cholesterol and reduces the amount of cholesterol the liver produces. So, by munching on plants we are doing some great things for our cholesterol levels.

Help lower blood pressure

Plant foods are brimming with supportive nutrients, such as antioxidants, vitamins, minerals and phytonutrients, which are supportive of heart health. Potassium, an important mineral found in many plants, such as sweet potatoes, bananas, spinach, avocados and black beans, is known to decrease blood pressure. It helps your body to get rid of sodium and eases pressure on blood vessels. Magnesium is also another important mineral that helps blood vessels relax to regulate blood pressure.

Provide fibre for your heart

High-fibre foods can lower blood pressure, cholesterol levels and inflammation, which in turn reduces the risk of hardening of the arteries, heart attacks and strokes. Scientists do not know exactly why this is the case but the research is compelling. Lab studies on human and animal cells show that the SCFAs (short-chain fatty acids) that fibre-rich foods break down into have a crucial role in lowering cholesterol, reducing fatty liver and minimising the risk of stroke. In one study of more than 40,000 male health professionals, those who ate lots of dietary fibre – especially cereal fibre – had a 40 per cent lower risk of coronary heart disease compared with men who ate the least fibre. Oats are one of my favourite breakfast foods because their soluble fibre reduces the amounts of LDL cholesterol circulating in the body. Add in some berries, seeds and nuts and you have a fibre-, antioxidant- and phytonutrient-rich start to the day which packs a powerful punch.

Slash your risk of cardiovascular disease

We know that lifestyle interventions can cut our risk of heart disease. Randomised control trials in nutrition are difficult to do accurately but there are a few notable studies that show us the power of plants when it comes to heart disease.

A DELVE INTO THE DATA

A lot of research in nutrition involves surveying large populations of people over time and asking them what they eat. This data can be used to notice who becomes ill. It is hard to do studies where participants have to actively change what they eat and this can only be done for short periods of time too. But these studies are useful, as they can test the observations that population studies make.

What do such studies show when it comes to heart disease? The Lyon diet heart study showed that a Mediterranean diet was good for heart health. The intervention group of cardiac patients were told to eat loads of fruit, vegetables, nuts, seeds and fish in place of meat and junk foods. They were able to demonstrate a 50–70 per cent reduced risk of a cardiovascular event.

Are there any studies looking at a plant-based diet and lifestyle interventions specifically? Yes, there are. These are smaller trials involving patients with heart disease who had already been given all that doctors had to offer. It would be wonderful to see these results repeated in larger trials with thousands of participants; hopefully researchers will do so, because the results are fascinating. The Lifestyle Heart Trial from 1990 involved 48 people who had already experienced heart attacks. They were advised to try a low-fat vegetarian diet, stop smoking and undergo stress management, as well as walking for 30 minutes every day. They were followed up for a year. Amazingly, the trial demonstrated for the first time a partial reversal of their clogged arteries. Not only that, but the patients lost weight and crucially experienced less angina pains than the control group. When patients were followed up five years later, those with arteries that were more than 50 per cent blocked had a nearly 8 per cent improvement in the blockages compared to a 27 per cent worsening in the blockages for those in the original control group. This shows that people were able to not only stick to a way of living that improved their angina, but also maintain the benefits they achieved during the study.

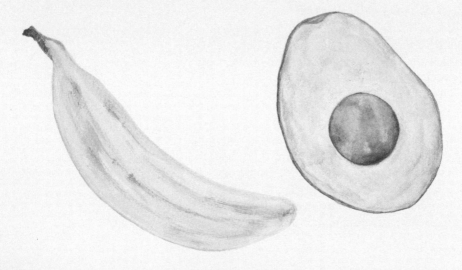

What about changing diet without exercise and stress management – could that help? Two studies by Dr Caldwell Esselstyn suggests that it could. Dr Esselstyn was able to help his trial participants achieve, with diet alone, improvement of plaques in severe heart disease. In 1985, he enlisted 22 end-stage heart-disease patients. These people had been sent home, having exhausted all medical therapies.

He advised them to eat a low-fat WFPB diet. Within 10 months of the start of treatment, a patient with severe right calf claudication (critically blocked arteries in his leg leading to severe pain on walking) experienced total pain relief and had measurably increased blood flow to his leg. This was so encouraging, he continued to follow up the small group of patients, adding in cholesterol lowering drugs as soon as they became available. He reported results after five and 12 years of follow-up. Of the 22 patients, 17 stuck with the diet and their disease progression halted.

Naturally, there is scepticism. That's not many people after all. Could it work more widely? Dr Esselstyn did a follow-up study in 2014 with nearly 200 people. These people were told to eat a WFPB diet as well as continue all their prescribed medical therapy.

What happened? Of the 198 patients with proven heart disease, 177 (89 per cent) stuck with the WFPB plan. There was one patient who had a stroke among them – a 0.6 per cent event rate.

Of the 21 people who didn't stick with the plan, 13 (62 per cent) had a cardiac event (a heart attack, stroke or bypass operation).

This is a huge difference. It suggests that the people who stopped eating a WFPB diet turned out to be one hundred times more likely to have a serious cardiac event.

The American College of Cardiology looked at a lot of data and released guidelines suggesting that a plant predominant diet is an integral tool to help prevent heart disease. A quote from their guidelines: 'A comparison of animal protein with plant protein . . . indicated that using meat for protein was associated with a 61 per cent increase in mortality rate, whereas replacing meat with nuts and seeds was associated with 40 per cent reduction in mortality rate.'

Why is this information useful? Because we can't always rely on medical procedures to fix us. What does all this mean? It means that even with established heart disease, there is hope that our food choices can help us. We have nothing to lose from adding healthy foods alongside all that modern medicine has to offer, and everything to gain.

A randomised controlled trial in the NEJM in 2007 showed that angiograms and stents do not prolong life in stable patients, and even bypass surgery was found to prolong life in less than 3 per cent of those who underwent surgery. Whereas according to the INTERHEART study, which followed 30,000 people over six continents, changing lifestyle could prevent the vast majority of all heart disease.

We should use everything we can – including cholesterol lowering drugs and procedures – to combat this disease. But it is also important to treat the underlying causes of heart disease, otherwise bypassed arteries will clog up again and eventually symptoms will return with a vengeance.

What will a WFPB diet do for you? Many of my patients say there is no point giving up something they enjoy unless they get something that they enjoy even more, and they want this outcome not years, but weeks later. I have found that the benefit of feeling better quickly is a very powerful motivator for my patients – and reframes goals from boring 'risk factor modification' to actual results for a happier, healthier life. In debates on disease prevention, doctors have often missed the point – our mortality rate is still always going to be 100 per cent. It's not just about how long we live, but how well we live. A WFPB lifestyle can improve quality of life for someone with angina very quickly, which is what helps these changes stick.

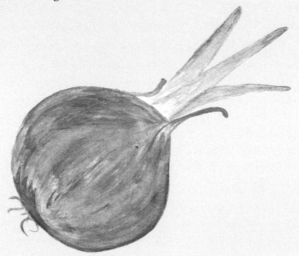

CASE STUDY – BRENDAN'S STORY

Brendan is a friend of mine and a huge inspiration.

A few days before Brendan's 37th birthday he felt an awkward shortness of breath while on his morning commute to work. Then it happened again on his way home. He realised how out of shape he must have got and vowed to start exercising again at some point. But the next day he became so short of breath he had to sit on a bench, his chest heaving. This was when he knew something wasn't right. He went to the doctor, who prescribed an antacid, an inhaler and arranged an ECG, which was normal. To be on the safe side, he was referred to a cardiologist for a stress test. He couldn't run on the treadmill or complete the test. He had a nuclear stress test instead, which uses a dye to directly measure the blood flow to the heart. Brendan's cardiologist looked at the reading and said, 'We need to get you to the emergency department – right now'.

Why the rush? One side of the screen was lit up like a Christmas tree and the other was blank. The blank screen meant there was no blood flowing to a large part of Brendan's heart – his LAD (left anterior descending) artery was completely blocked. This is known as the widow maker; he was at risk of a fatal heart attack unless he had a procedure to immediately open up this vessel and allow blood to flow. His head was spinning – he was only 37 years old and he could drop dead at any moment? He was scared but agreed to surgery. The next morning, he had a stent inserted to open up the blood flow and his pain and shortness of breath melted away.

But the thought still nagged at him – what if this was to happen again? What if the stent blocked up? A doctor had mentioned a Mediterranean diet – would that help? He decided to re-watch the documentary film, *Forks Over Knives*. A doctor friend had taken him to see it years before, but after his brush with death, he decided to watch it again. The film explains the heart health benefits of a plant-based diet. The chicken he was served in his hospital bed was the last piece of meat he ate. He bought a Vitamix on his way home from hospital. He began to take control of his health and he felt that 'finally I had hope, and a path out of my current situation'.

Brendan underwent an intensive three-month programme at his local Cardiac Rehabilitation Centre. He was the youngest person in the room by a generation.

'I remember walking in, so scared I was going to drop dead on a treadmill. I walked slower than molasses and was winded by the time the first session was complete.'

But, he did it and was ready for more. Slowly Brendan built his confidence and over time he was able to jog on the treadmill. He lost weight, felt fantastic and by the time he had finished the cardiac rehabilitation programme he was running five miles at a time and had lost three and a half stone in three months.

'I was light on my feet and full of energy thanks to the plant-based lifestyle I had started. Each day I grew more aware of the mind–body connection and my relationship with not only food but myself began to improve.'

Almost three years after Brendan's heart procedure, he finished the Atlantic City Ironman 70.3 and went on to complete the NYC Marathon in 2019.

When I asked him how he felt about his experiences, he said, 'I could not be more grateful for this entire experience. I feel the once forgotten person I lost years ago is coming back; now I am focused and driven to live a long, healthy, impactful and meaningful life – fuelled by plants!'

HOW FAT INFLUENCES OUR HEALTH

Low fat? More fat? Zero fat? What is the best for our bodies? Fat gets a bad rap. For years we have been told that fat will make us pile on the pounds, raise our cholesterol and lead to health issues. But we all need a regular amount of fat to give us energy, help us absorb vital nutrients and protect our organs. 'Bad' fats are responsible for all the things that fats are blamed for, including clogged arteries and increased risk of heart disease, whereas 'good fats', such as unsaturated fats and omega-3s have the opposite effect and can lower the risk of heart disease.

To understand more about the role fats play in a healthy diet, it is a good idea to look at the main types of fat: saturated, unsaturated and trans fat. Remember: Not all fats are created equal.

SATURATED FAT

This type of fat comes mainly from animal sources, such as red meat, poultry and full-fat dairy products. It is linked with high cholesterol levels and increased risk of heart disease and also contains a lot of calories. Saturated fat can sometimes occur in some non-animal foods, such as coconut oil and palm oil. The NHS recommends that men have no more than 30g saturated fat a day, women no more than 20g saturated fat a day and that children should have less. Eating foods with too much saturated fat in them changes the way our liver processes cholesterol. Our livers have LDL receptors in them and when LDL cholesterol passes through, the receptor takes it out of the blood to be broken down – these receptors are 'in charge'. However, having too much cholesterol in the diet can stop these receptors from working well. This is one of many reasons to reduce animal foods and junk foods, to improve the way our liver functions too.

TRANS FAT

Trans fat (or trans fatty acids), only makes up 0.8 per cent
of the average UK diet, but it is considered the most harmful
fat. It is a form of processed cooking oil and can be found in
doughnuts, fast food and other products like some margarines.
Small amounts can also be found naturally in meat. In 2012, in
the UK, most supermarkets and large fast-food chains signed a
voluntary agreement to not use artificial trans fats and while the UK
government has urged food companies to cut down the level of trans
fats in products, an outright ban has not yet been enforced. It is not
entirely clear how many products still contain them. Trans fats are
known to raise cholesterol and to increase the risk of developing
heart disease and a number of other chronic illnesses, including
Type 2 diabetes and Alzheimer's. So, although far less common
now, try to limit your intake of processed foods to reduce the risk of
exposure to trans fats.

UNSATURATED FAT

Unsaturated fats are better for us and consist of monounsaturated
fatty acids (MUFAs) and polyunsaturated fatty acids (PUFAs).
Polyunsaturated fats include ALA (alpha-linolenic acid) and LA
(linoleic acid) which are the 'parent fats' that make omega-3 and
omega-6 fats respectively. These parent fats are essential because
they cannot be made by the body. Generally, seeds are rich in PUFAs
and nuts are rich in MUFAs. Long-chain omega-3 fats (DHA and
EPA) are made in the body by using the parent fat ALA, but in a lot
of people this process can be inefficient. The body can perform this
conversion better when there are more omega-3 fats in the diet, so
limiting saturated fats from junk food and omega-6-rich oils, such as
sunflower oil, helps. DHA and EPA can also be found ready made in
fish, and in the algae that fish eat. This is why people who avoid fish
are often advised to consider algae oil supplements. This is a way of
going direct to source, where the fish get their EPA and DHA from,
and is also more environmentally friendly than eating fish.

The important thing to remember is that by replacing saturated
fats with unsaturated fats (MUFAs and PUFAs), we can improve
our health and reduce our cholesterol and heart disease risk. These
'good' fats are found in a plethora of delicious foods, including
seeds, such as chia, flax and hemp seeds. A tablespoon of ground
flax seeds a day is my top tip for getting a decent plant-based

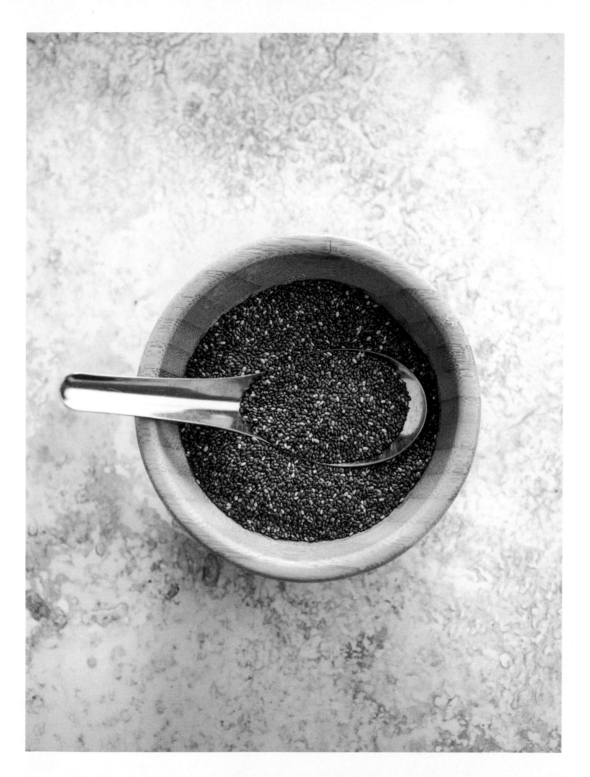

omega-3; you can sprinkle it onto cereal, porridge or yoghurt, use it as an egg substitute in baking, or mixed into a curry or stew.

As well as a great source of protein, some nuts – including almonds, Brazils and peanuts – are also packed with monounsaturated fatty acids. So, try to include these in your food shop every week.

Oily fish are a source of these healthy omega-3 fats. However, they also contain saturated fat and no fibre. Unfortunately, they also now contain the toxins (POPs – persistent organic pollutants) and microplastics we have let into the ocean. Tiny pieces of degraded plastic, synthetic fibres and plastic beads have become a common feature of sea life now. These particles can compromise the immune function and reproductive health of fish. Crucially, both microplastics and chemicals can accumulate up the food chain, affecting us too. This means fish is no longer the obvious healthy choice it used to be, and is not included in a WFPB diet.

When it comes to fish, let's also look at the whole picture. According to many scientists, world fish stocks will collapse by 2050 at current use and levels of sea warming. This suggests we will have to move away from eating fish regularly; it will be inevitable in the coming years. The good news is that we can choose plant-based omega-3s (e.g. flax seeds, chia seeds and walnuts) or an algae-based EPA/DHA supplement instead.

WHICH FATS SHOULD WE EAT?

Now you know what each of the fats are, enjoy whole plant foods that happen to contain healthful fats such as nuts, seeds and avocados along with a wide range of plant foods to ensure you are 'eating a rainbow'.

Limit foods that contain unhealthful saturated fats such as pastries, battered foods, fried foods and animal products and instead enjoy wholefoods like flax seeds and nuts, as opposed to refined, liquid oils. For more recommendations about how much fat to consume, see the 'Eat Well Guide' (page 142).

For some people, oils can trigger inflammatory arthritis pains. Low-oil and oil-free diets have been used to improve heart disease too. If either condition is a cause of concern for you, limit your oil intake. However, extra virgin olive oil has been found to be heart healthy, containing antioxidants and MUFAs, which is good news for those of us who like a drizzle of extra virgin olive oil on our salads. For inspiration on wholefoods plant-based and oil-free cooking methods, see the recipe section (pages 190–265).

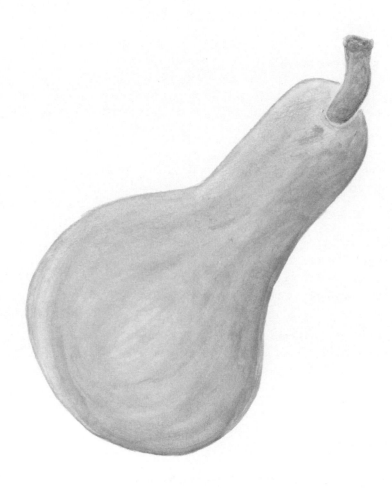

RETHINKING CANCER

First, the bad news. Cancer is one of the leading causes of premature death in the UK and by that, I mean death before the age of 75. Despite the many millions of pounds that have been spent on research, cancer remains the second biggest cause of death in the Western world. One in two people born after 1960 will develop cancer. In my surgery, I see many people who are living with cancer of all forms and I feel that it is something we all struggle to think about if we are not affected by it. We all think it won't happen to us.

All of our lives are touched by cancer. It is highly likely that you know or love someone who has had cancer and, perhaps as you read this, you have cancer yourself. There is no doubt that the 'C' word strikes fear into many of my patients and it is one of the hardest things to have to share when breaking bad news.

My patients who have been diagnosed with cancer have often told me that they feel helpless in so many ways. Sometimes they even feel that it is their fault. Let me be clear: there is never any blame when a cancer diagnosis occurs. People with the healthiest of lifestyles and the lowest risk can sometimes develop cancer.

When you have cancer, in essence, something has caused an imbalance in the way the body 'sees' itself, making cells unable to communicate with each other to allow programmed cell death when it is needed. So, the confused cell does the only thing it knows how to and multiplies to survive.

We can never fully know 'why' this happens, but there are a few things we can say for sure. Our genes directly contribute to about 10 per cent of cancers and this is something we cannot control. However, for most of us, we do have the potential to make important changes to our lifestyle to reduce the risk of cancer.

Do we start with diet? After all, food is the main building block we use to create our body, cancer cells and all. When it comes to the food we eat, there is no single superfood to prevent cancer. Looking at populations for clues is interesting. What we see is that the global transition from rural, fresh and vegetable-rich diets to one with more animal products and processed foods with increased sugar and fat may account for much of the increase in the disease.

When it comes to research into cancer and diet, the waters are muddy. This is because people don't eat exactly same foods throughout their lifetimes, and it can be hard to unpick which habits they have that pose the largest risk. We can look at specific substances or foods under the microscope and say whether there is a plausible reason why they may cause cancer cells to multiply. However, the kinds of trials drug companies often use to test whether a new medicine will work can't easily be done when it comes to nutrition.

We can piece together a few things based on different kinds of research that look at lifestyle patterns, the mechanisms that cause cancer and testing diets and interventions to see what makes an impact. When each of these kinds of research point to similar things we can say with some confidence we have found a piece of advice that sticks. The scientific term for looking at lots of data sets together is a meta-analysis.

LAB LESSONS

Do we know what substances cause cancer? Asbestos is an obvious one. Benzene from coal tar is another, and can be inhaled from petrol stations, cigarettes, car exhausts, glue, paints and detergents. Exposure to benzenes has been linked to blood cancers like leukaemia and has also been found to affect fertility.

One of the main carcinogens we don't really think about comes from alcohol – acetaldehyde. This is the first and most toxic metabolite from alcohol and reacts with our DNA to form cancer-promoting compounds. Lab studies on animals, as well as population data shows this to be the case. It is an uncomfortable truth, as alcohol is so ingrained in Western cultures and has been a way of celebrating, socialising and consoling for generations. However, understanding this information and choosing to apply it – or choosing not to – should be a decision we can make with facts as well as our emotions and habits.

Awareness is key, as I find moderation means different things to different people. I had one patient convinced that drinking two litres of cider a day was normal. Knowledge can be important in changing how we feel about the things we enjoy.

There are some chemicals derived from foods that have been shown to be cancer causing. Heterocyclic amines (HCAs) are formed in animal proteins that are cooked at high temperature, such as over an open flame. You know those charred blackened lines on your barbecued burger? HCAs are highest in pan-fried and barbecued meats and can be in lower concentration when meat is poached or stewed. There are no HCAs produced when you barbecue vegetables. A specific HCA that has been studied a lot is PhIP. A study of over 29,000 men from 2005 identified PhIP from cooked meat as a likely factor in the increased rates of prostate cancer in the men participating in the study. Another intriguing study also links the presence of PhIP to breast cancer – the researchers took breast tissue from women undergoing breast reduction surgery, so the breast surgery had nothing to do with cancer, and interviewed them about their diet. The breast tissue was analysed for the presence of DNA adducts – the bits of DNA bound to carcinogens which are early marker of cancerous change. They found that fried meat, beef and processed meats in the diet were all associated with pre-cancerous changes in the breast tissue that was removed from these women.

There are other products of cooking meat at high temperature that are potential carcinogens as well, including polycyclic aromatic hydrocarbons (PAHs) and advanced glycation end products (AGEs).

Acrylamide is a carcinogen that occurs when oils with low smoke points are heated. Think French fries, potato crisps and burned toast. This is why using oils with high smoke points is better for cooking (cold-pressed canola oil and avocado oil for example) or using no-oil cooking techniques as discussed in the recipe section. I know none of us wants to hear that beer and barbecues are bad for us – but the good news is that eating vegetables can do a lot to offset the damage caused by these compounds. Studies show eating fruits and veggies can block these carcinogenic compounds, with studies highlighting the moderate ability of black, green and rooibos tea as well as cherry, spinach and onion juices to block these compounds. Whatever stage you are at with your health, it is never too late to take advantage of vegetables and their protective compounds for your well-being.

HORMONES AND CANCER

What else has been shown to increase cancer risk? High levels of the hormones insulin and IGF-1 (insulin like growth factor 1). This is particularly a problem for people who are overweight or living with insulin resistance and Type 2 diabetes. IGF-1 is a growth hormone we make in our bodies and it is important for helping us grow new tissue. But like all hormones, you need to have just the right amount. IGF-1 is produced by the liver and is highest in childhood (for growth) and naturally declines in adulthood. But we now know that IGF-1 also promotes each of the key stages of cancer development: growth of the cancerous cells, vascularisation of cancerous tissue (blood vessel growth) and metastasis (spread). Eating animal products causes our bodies to produce more IGF-1 than we need. IGF-1 is known to be a risk factor for bowel cancer, where the foods we eat interact directly with the gut lining. Population studies show us that increased IGF-1 is linked to increased prostate cancer. In fact, the strength of the IGF-1 and prostate cancer link is considerable. According to one study, it has the same level of importance as the association between high blood lipid levels and heart disease.

Restricting energy (fasting) and restricting animal protein causes IGF-1 levels to fall to normal in animal studies. Most people are reluctant to undergo a 'mild starvation' diet to boost lifespan and it can be hard to sustain over time. The good news is that in humans, restricting animal protein alone seems to be better at reducing IGF-1 than severe calorie restriction. This means you can get great benefits from maximising your plant proteins without having to go hungry.

Oestrogen is another key player in the development of hormone-linked cancers such as breast, ovarian and prostate. Our bodies produce more oestrogen in certain types of fat cell, which may be why obesity is linked with a higher risk of certain cancers. But could the oestrogen in our food and drink play a part? Research on this is mixed. What we can say for sure is that cow's milk contains more oestrogen than it used to, given that cows are pregnant at the same time as lactating nowadays, and pregnancy increases oestrogen levels in all mammals.

Certain types of plastics are also known to be hormone disruptors which can mimic oestrogen in our bodies. So, drinking cow's milk from a plastic bottle could reasonably increase the amount of oestrogen your body is exposed to.

HAEM IRON

Iron is a crucial mineral for cell proliferation and growth. Haem iron from meat is much easier to absorb, which is really helpful if you are anaemic. But the body has no way of regulating its absorption of haem iron and haem iron also oxidises easily (a bit like the rust you see on a car, or the brown of an apple after it has been exposed to the air). When oxidation happens in the body it can lead to oxidative stress (see page 30), which, as we discussed earlier, can accelerate the ageing process.

Haem iron has also been found to cause the formation of N-nitroso compounds (NOC) in the body, which damage the cells that line the bowel and contribute to bowel cancer. One study showed that supplementation with haem iron spiked NOC levels, whereas iron-rich plant sources did not. It also showed that eating meat increased NOC in stools, whereas veggie iron sources did not.

Eating lentils and beans will give you iron in a way that does not increase your cancer risk, as well as an abundance of fibre, plant protein and phytochemicals. My favourite iron-rich foods include legumes, seeds, nuts, dates and quinoa. Having said that, plant foods do not let go of their iron as easily, as it is bound to substances called phytates and oxalates. You can maximise your absorption of iron by pairing vitamin C-rich foods with your beans and wholegrains (like squeezing lemon juice on your curry) and avoiding tea and coffee with your meals (which contain tannins that have been found to reduce the amount of iron the body can absorb).

DOES THIS MEAN MEAT IS OFF THE MENU?

The World Health Organization was tasked with looking at a whole bunch of studies to come up with a global, rational consensus as to whether the balance of evidence could say what the risks are. They analysed over 800 different studies of cancer. The result?

They found bacon, sausages, ham, salami and other processed meats to be 'group 1' carcinogens. This means that these substances are known to cause cancer. The level of risk of group 1 substances are not all the same (for example, smoking and asbestos exposure is considered a higher risk) but the risks from processed red meats cannot be ignored. Red meats, such as beef, lamb and pork have been classified as Group 2A carcinogens, which means that they probably cause cancer.

The Scientific Advisory Committee on Nutrition (SACN) produced a report in 2010 called 'Iron and Health' that influenced UK dietary guidelines. The report could not identify the amount of red or processed meat which might increase the risk of cancer, so sensibly the advice was to cut down. Based on the average man eating about 88g red meat a day, the suggestion was to reduce this amount to 70g. This also fits with the average daily maximum suggested by the WHO.

As a visual guide, a thin slice of ham is about 23g and an average pork sausage weighs about 75g, which is already over the daily maximum allowance.

If you can't imagine giving up meat, consider reducing your intake so you are not eating it every day. Try opting for the WFPB diet most of the time and really enjoy a good-quality (small) portion of meat within the guidelines above. Think of it as a 'condimeat', rather than the main event. I would always encourage you to enjoy a WFPB diet as far as possible to reap the most benefits.

Alongside understanding the impact meat has on our health, we are becoming much more aware as a society of the environmental impact of the intensive breeding of livestock. The damage that their waste products does to our water systems, the inefficient use of land (for growing food that goes to the animals and not to people), and the long-term risks when antibiotics are used to treat animals who become unwell when living in cramped conditions.

When we eat animals that have been treated with antibiotics, we may also increase our own risk of antibiotic resistance. We need antibiotics to work when we get ill. In addition, there are studies that show that antibiotics deplete our gut bacteria, which in turn increases our risk of getting certain forms of cancer.

Do not be dismayed by this section if you have lived most of your life eating meat. Most of us have. As you consider your future health, I hope this section gives you that extra little nudge towards trying a plant-based alternative to give your body the best chance of a cancer-free future.

HOW PLANTS CAN HELP

The World Cancer Research Fund tells us to maximise fruits, vegetables, wholegrains and pulses in our diets to prevent cancer. What do we know about vegetarian or vegan diets and cancer? Let's look at two long-term studies to help us. The Adventist Health Study-2 explores the links between lifestyle, diet and disease outcomes, and includes more than 96,000 people from the Seventh Day Adventist Community from North America. The EPIC-Oxford Study has similar aims and includes more than 65,000 people from the UK. The Adventist Health Study-2 began in 2002 and the EPIC-Oxford study started in 1993 and both of these studies are ongoing. These studies are by no means perfect, but they help us to look at overall eating patterns. Vegans in these groups are probably closest to a WFPB lifestyle of all groups studied, especially in the Adventist population study data.

In both studies, around a quarter to a third of participants are vegan or vegetarian. In the Adventist Health Study 2, vegans have a 16 per cent reduced risk of cancer and the vegetarians have an 8 per cent reduced risk of cancer. In the EPIC-Oxford study, vegans have a 19 per cent reduced risk of cancer and the vegetarians have an 11 per cent reduced risk of cancer. We can therefore begin to see that what we choose to eat plays a role in the prevention and development of this disease.

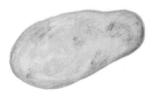 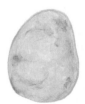 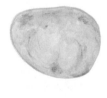

HOW CAN WE ASSESS THE IMPACT OF PLANT FOODS ON REDUCING CANCER RISK?

Research into which foods are more carcinogenic is useful, in that it allows us to analyse associations between diet and health outcomes, but researchers wanted to go a step further and so developed the Plant-Based Diet Index, a scoring system to assess the impact of healthy plant foods on developing cancer and other chronic diseases. This system gives positive marks for consumption of fruits, vegetables, wholegrains, nuts, tea and coffee and vegetable oils. Negative scores are given for fruit juice, refined grains, potatoes (perhaps because they are often fried as chips and crisps), sugar-sweetened beverages, sweets and desserts. All animal foods, including meat, fish and dairy, are given negative scores. The Nutrinet-Sante Cohort Study followed more than 54,000 people over four years. People with high scores on the Plant-Based Diet Index had a 15 per cent reduced cancer risk and there was a particular benefit seen for reducing the risk of colorectal and lung cancers.

WHY ARE PLANTS SO GREAT AT REDUCING CANCER RISK?

A WFPB diet is:

Rich in nutrients, including antioxidants and phytochemicals that can reduce oxidative stress and inflammation.

Low in calories, which can help to maintain a healthy BMI.

High in fibre that is good for our microbiome, which is important for boosting immunity.

Free of the majority of carcinogens

Good for maintaining hormone balance

There are many bioactive compounds in fruit and vegetables that are thought to prevent, delay and help destroy cancer cells. Cruciferous vegetables are particularly well known for their cancer-defying properties. Think kale, broccoli, cress, cauliflower and sprouts. They are packed with nutrients, such as the carotenoids lutein and carotene, vitamins C, E and beta-carotene, folate, minerals and plenty of fibre. They also contain a group of compounds

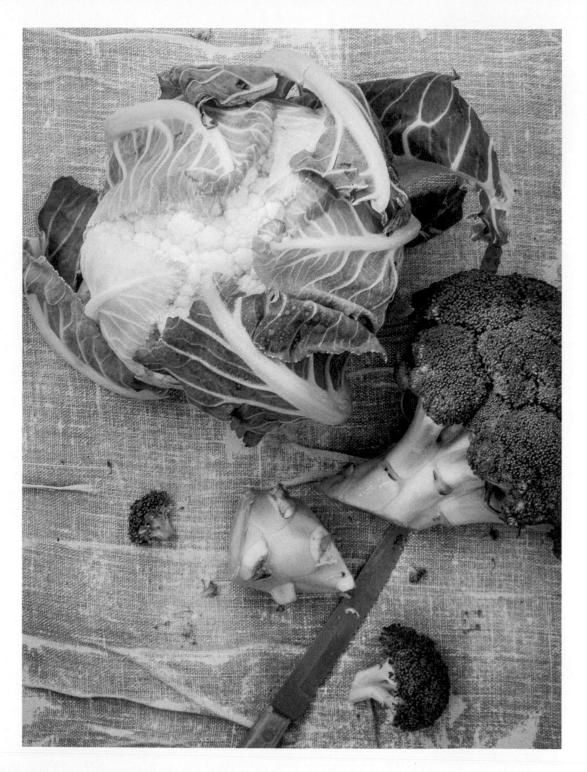

THE PLANT POWER DOCTOR

called glucosinolates, which are responsible for the bitter taste and flavour of these vegetables, and are associated with decreased inflammation and improved liver health. Studies have found strong links between greater consumption of cruciferous vegetables and reduced risk of lung, breast, prostate, colorectal and other cancers. More recent studies have concluded that the compounds found in cruciferous vegetables 'turn on' genes that slow tumour growth, and stimulate self-destruction of cancer cells, a process called apoptosis. In addition, glucosinolates may also stimulate enzymes that deactivate carcinogens and decrease cancer cells' ability to spread. Interestingly, although these compounds are not degraded by cooking, the enzymes that turn them into active compounds are. The answer? Eating them raw is one option. Another is to chop the veggies and leave them for 40 minutes or so. The act of chopping or chewing will provide the enzymes with enough time to work before the vegetables are cooked. This is known as the 'hack 'n' hold' technique. Think about this tonight when making your dinner; you can chop the veggies earlier to give yourself even more benefits.

Flavonoids are a large family of phytonutrients, of which thousands have been identified. Examples include apigenin, baicalein, luteolin and rutin. There is no reason to doubt that many more thousands of such compounds may exist. The amazing thing is that these nutrients cannot simply be extracted and expected to have the same health benefits. In fact, vitamin supplements in excess have in some cases been found to be actively harmful. The point here is that real plant foods, eaten close to how they were grown in nature, seem to have a synergistic effect on health which is impossible to replicate in pill form. Much as we try, we just cannot clump together amino acids, vitamins and fibre in the same way that nature can.

FIBRE

Fibre sweeps up any waste along our intestine, including getting rid of carcinogens before they can become an issue, and it is even thought that fibre may change these cancer-causing compounds so they are less harmful. But the fibre has to work with our beneficial gut bugs in order to reap the most rewards. Good bacteria in the colon ferment fibre into short-chain fatty acids (SCFAs), which are healthy fuel for the cells in our gut lining. These amazing compounds (butyrate, proprionate and acetate) reduce the likelihood that the cells in the intestine will become cancerous. Lab studies show that butyrate helps keep colon cells healthy, prevents the growth of tumour cells and encourages cancer cell destruction in the colon. Many population studies have also linked high-fibre diets to reduced risk of colon cancer.

It has also been found that as well as colorectal cancer, fibre plays a role in reducing the risk of other types of cancer. One study found that women who consumed a higher amount of fibre reduce their lifetime risk of developing breast cancer by 12 per cent. So instead of having a chicken salad or a lamb curry tomorrow, you could switch to a bean salad or a chickpea curry to improve your fibre intake.

WHAT ROLE DOES DIET PLAY IN CANCER TREATMENT?

There is still much research to be done in this area but we do know that following a WFPB diet has benefits alongside traditional treatment pathways. Good nutrition in general can play an important role in coping with cancer and chemotherapy side effects. I recognise that a cancer diagnosis is a time of great stress and uncertainty. Do not put extra stress on yourself over what you are eating. This is a challenging time and it is important to be kind to yourself. It is also important to remember that what you eat is not an alternative to the medicines and treatments that your specialists have recommended, but can be used alongside them to help you, if and when you feel ready to approach it.

For people who already have a cancer diagnosis, it has been shown that a high intake of fruit and vegetables could improve prognosis. The Women's Intervention Nutrition Study (WINS) showed that women who had been diagnosed with breast cancer tended to live longer without relapse when they reduced their fat intake, which is generally linked with reduced consumption of animal foods. Sometimes eating can become difficult due to the side effects from cancer. However, good nutrition can help people to maintain weight and energy, help with tolerating treatment-related side effects, and promote healing and faster recovery from sometimes gruelling courses of chemotherapy. Researchers have demonstrated that apigenin, which is found in fruit (including apples, cherries and grapes), vegetables (including artichokes and celery), herbs (including parsley and basil), nuts and some teas has been shown to have potential anti-tumour effects in several kinds of cancer.

Another of the cancer-busting mechanisms of fruit and vegetables is the ability of plants to inhibit the ironically named 'VEGF', which stands for vascular endothelial growth factor. VEGF reduces the ability of tumours to obtain a reliable blood supply, which they need in order to grow. The formation of new blood vessels, called 'angiogenesis' also plays a central role in the progression of solid tumours, including those of the lung, colon, bladder, breast, cervix and prostate. If there is no VEGF, the blood vessels tumours need to support their growth will not be able to form. What compounds in fruit may be responsible for helping to prevent the action of VEGF? Resveratrol which is found in grape skin and berries inhibits VEGF and blood vessel growth in tumours. Berries also contain high concentrations of proanthocyanidin, another compound that can suppress cancer growth.

What does all this mean? No one can promise that food can treat cancer. That would be irresponsible. No one can tell you how much you would need to eat to benefit either. This is not easy to know. But gaining some insight from these studies can help you to make food choices that help you in your cancer journey. Enjoying berries and grapes every day not only tastes great, but can be a great tool for improving your health if you are living with cancer.

WHAT ELSE CAN YOU DO TO LOWER YOUR RISK OF CANCER?

The World Cancer Research Fund and the American Institute for Cancer Research have created a report with no government or industry ties. The expert panel reviewed nearly a thousand papers over three years and unanimously agreed on these main points – ten key recommendations for us that could be the difference between having cancer and avoiding it. These recommendations are in addition to avoiding smoking and unsafe sun exposure.

- Be a healthy weight.
- Be physically active as part of everyday life.
- Eat a diet rich in wholegrains, vegetables, fruit and beans.
- Limit consumption of 'fast foods' and other processed foods high in fat, salt or sugars.
- Limit consumption of red meat and avoid processed meat.
- Limit consumption of sugar-sweetened drinks.

- Limit alcoholic drinks.

- Do not use supplements for cancer prevention – aim to meet nutritional needs through your food where possible.

- For mothers, breastfeed your baby, if you can.

- After a cancer diagnosis: follow our recommendations if you can.

Highly processed foods that are packed with sugar and low in fibre are on this list and linked to cancer. One study looking at the medical records and eating habits of over 100,000 adults, showed that every 10 per cent increase in ultra-processed foods that they ate was linked to a 10 per cent increase in risk for certain cancers. I feel that these foods should have health warnings like cigarette packets now do. Otherwise people have no idea how to quantify the risk they are taking by eating these accessible and comforting foods every day.

One study looked at data from both the Nurses' Health Study and the Health Professionals Follow-Up Study to answer the question of what habits increase cancer risk. It examined five major risk factors in participants: whether they had ever smoked; whether they exercised regularly; whether they consumed low amounts of alcohol; whether they were a healthy weight; and the quality of their diet. The diet looked at a high intake of fruit, vegetables, wholegrains, unsaturated fats and omega-3 fats, with a low intake of red and processed meats, sugar-sweetened drinks, trans fats and salt. The results showed that those who had the best diet scores had a 30 per cent reduced risk of dying from cancer. But those who had all five lifestyle factors under control had a 65 per cent reduced risk of death from cancer.

EXERCISE

So, we know cancer risk is about so much more than food alone. It is also about the bigger picture when it comes to lifestyle. For example, one study involving over 405,000 men and women in Taiwan looked at the combined effect of eight common chronic disease markers on cancer risk compared to other lifestyle factors. Interestingly, they found that there was nearly a 40 per cent reduction in excess risks of cancer and cancer deaths for people who exercised regularly. Lack of exercise in our life should be an important part of the discussion on cancer prevention.

SLEEP

Lack of sleep is important too. In October 2007, the International Agency for Research on Cancer (IARC) classified shift work with sleep-wake cycle disruption as a probable human carcinogen. Light during the 'biological night' disturbs the circadian system, alters sleep-activity patterns (including when we eat and the efficiency of our digestion), suppresses melatonin production, and wreaks havoc on the circadian genes for cancer-related pathways in the body. This is another reason why smartphones and TV should ideally be limited at night.

EMR

Could there be another reason to limit our exposure to devices? Some animal studies show increased DNA oxidation when the animals are exposed to typical amounts of electromagnetic radiation as would be emitted from a mobile phone. Case control studies show an association between long-term mobile phone use and malignant brain tumours, among others. We are surrounded by these frequencies, from wireless headphones to smartphones, from smart meters to smart watches and domestic appliances. The IARC classify radiofrequency electromagnetic radiation as a group 2B carcinogen, meaning it is possibly cancer causing.

More studies are needed, as animal studies and case control studies are simply not evidence enough to say with certainty whether there is an effect on humans from being surrounded by wireless technology, or not. Non-ionising radiation is often thought of as harmless, as it is not very strong, and it does not burn like excess sun might. But some scientists have been concerned about the high level of pulsations that a higher frequency such as 5G uses, which could be more biologically active. A European Parliament report (from the EPRS) published in March 2020 concluded more research was needed and called for coordinated efforts by physicists, engineers and medics to understand if there is a potential risk to human health worth understanding. Until more is known, I feel a precautionary principle is worth taking. What would that look like in practical terms? Perhaps switching off your Wi-Fi at night, limiting your time with your phone in your pocket or next to your head, and also reducing your children's exposure to devices as much as is practically possible in this age of wireless technology. There is no harm in being cautious until we have a larger collective body of research available to show us that caution is no longer required.

STRESS

Lastly, I feel it is also crucial to touch upon the role of stress. Clinical studies over the past 30 years have provided strong evidence for links between chronic stress, depression and social isolation and the progression of cancer. In breast cancer patients, social support has been related to longer survival in several large-scale studies. And when we look at the outcome of stress on our bodies, it is easy to see why. Stress hormones stimulate angiogenesis, cell migration and invasion, and can therefore lead to increased tumour growth and progression whereas feel-good hormones such as dopamine can inhibit this process. What can we learn from this? Sometimes, laughter and love truly are the best medicine. When cancer becomes such a fear-inducing prospect, our bodies need hope and happiness just as much as a good diet, exercise and sleep.

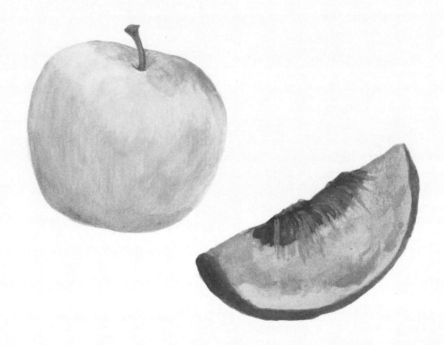

CASE STUDY – EM'S STORY

In December 2018, 30-year old Em noticed a lump in her breast and a few days later, she noticed some blood discharging from one of her nipples. She was young and had no family history of breast cancer, so she was not too concerned. Despite her initial lack of fear, during her scan the radiology doctor who did an ultrasound and took the biopsies, had seen enough for him to break from the usual protocol. He informed her that ultrasound scan was strongly suggestive of breast cancer.

After weeks of tests, it was confirmed Em had Stage 4 breast cancer and it had spread: she had a 10cm tumour in her breast, numerous tumours in her armpit, five tumours in her liver, a tumour in her spine and one in her neck. It was on this day that her world turned upside down. Her oncologist wanted to make sure that she understood the severity of the situation and explained that she was considered palliative and that the aim of treatment was to prolong her life rather than to cure the cancer. He went on to tell her that the average survival is just three and a half years and there is no cure. Her daughter was just a year old. Em is a doctor specialising in mental health, and this figure deeply shocked her.

'My soul was crushed and all I could think about was my daughter having to grow up without a mum, and my poor husband having to raise her alone,' Em said. 'After leaving that appointment I felt that I could drop dead at any moment.

'I went on to experience a period of grief, I was mourning the loss of the life that I thought I would live. This was a difficult period of time, but I managed to get through it, and when I emerged from the other side, I was a different person.'

Em hung onto the fact that for unknown reasons a small minority of people do go on to live long lives, so she knew that it was possible for her to outlive the prognosis. She also knew from what her oncologist had said that the solution to her problem wasn't necessarily within the bounds of conventional modern medicine.

After doing her own research she became aware of the fact that regular exercise and maintaining a healthy weight were associated with better breast cancer outcomes, so she was keen to make a start with these changes. After her research, she also switched from a standard Western diet consuming meat and dairy regularly to a completely WFPB diet and took steps to manage her stress levels, such as prioritising sleep and rest. Above all, she wanted to bring more joy and laughter into her life and wanted to bring the fun back into relaxation and stress management.

She is now around 18 months post-diagnosis and incredibly her most recent scans have showed no evidence of cancer.

She said: 'Can I tell you exactly how this has been achieved? No. But what I can tell you is that many people have been on the exact same oral chemotherapy and hormone treatment as me and many of these people have not experienced such miracles. I do not for one second want to blow my own trumpet or make out that I am special, but what I would like to do is to make you feel empowered. I would like to let you know that when it comes to your health, you are not powerless, and the labels that doctors may give you do not need to define you. Food is medicine, laughter is medicine, movement is medicine and human connection is also most certainly medicine.'

While one person's story cannot apply to everyone, the scientific evidence discussed in this chapter certainly suggests that for Em, and for many others, lifestyle changes, healthy foods, stressing less, loving more and moving your body will help when dealing with cancer and its effects.

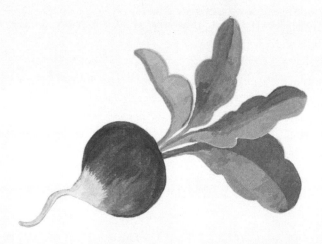

DIABETES DISCOVERIES

Diabetes is now a global health issue. More people than ever before have diabetes, and if nothing changes, more than 5 million people will have diabetes in the UK by 2025 (at the time of writing it is thought that 4.7 million people in the UK have diabetes and someone is diagnosed every three minutes).

Heart disease is the biggest cause of premature death for diabetics, and 80 per cent of people living with diabetes will die of a heart attack or a stroke. Before this they can suffer problems with their vision, their digestion and even their ability to have a sexual relationship with their partner. The good news is that much of this can be prevented.

Around 90 per cent of people with diabetes have Type 2 diabetes – and although the tendency to Type 2 diabetes runs in families, it can usually be prevented through our lifestyles. The dramatic increase in obesity is the main reason there are so many more people living with Type 2 diabetes today than there were just 20 years ago. In 1996 there were only 1.4 million people diagnosed with diabetes, and young people being affected was almost unheard of. Today, it is a different story. Yes, our increasing size is an important factor in increasing the risk of diabetes, but there are many other contributors, including a disrupted gut microbiome, poor sleep, exercising less and chronic stress. All of these factors play a part.

All types of diabetes have one thing in common – they cause people to have too much sugar in the form of glucose in their blood. Glucose is formed when the body breaks down the carbohydrates that we eat or drink. The glucose is then released into the blood. Glucose is important because it is a precious fuel for all the cells in our body, gives us energy to move our muscles, and is the brain's preferred energy source. But it needs to get into our cells, not stay in the bloodstream. High levels of glucose that stay in the blood circulation can act like a toxin, damaging nerves and organs that the blood reaches.

The glucose gets inside our cells with the help of insulin. Insulin is our fantastic transporter hormone. It transports fats, proteins and most importantly glucose around the body. It is made in the beta cells of the pancreas and acts like a key in a lock by attaching to little channels on the cell membrane. This opens the channel – or receptor – in the cell to let glucose in. If there is not enough insulin being made, the glucose travelling around the bloodstream cannot get into the cells where it is needed and is stuck in the blood vessels where it can cause damage. This happens in Type 1 Diabetes.

With Type 2 diabetes, the problem is with a jammed lock, or a receptor that is not functioning normally. If the lock on the cell membrane is jammed, the insulin keys our body makes cannot unlock the cell receptor and let glucose in. This is also called 'insulin resistance'. The pancreas then tries to make more insulin, or more keys to use on the jammed lock. But making more keys doesn't fix the lock and results in higher levels of both insulin and glucose in the blood, both of which can be harmful in excess.

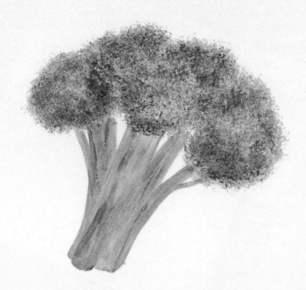

DIABETES EXPLAINED

Type 1 diabetes

Type 1 diabetes happens when the body stops making insulin. This is because the cells where insulin is made (pancreatic beta cells) have been destroyed, usually by the body's own immune system. Some of us have specific genetic risks, and then an environmental trigger switches those genes on, causing the autoimmune response. Sometimes this could be a virus, or a trauma, and some studies even point to cow's milk protein exposures in susceptible people. When the body is no longer able to use insulin to transport glucose, fatty acids or proteins, it will shut down fast. That's why without insulin injections, Type 1 diabetics would not be able to survive for very long.

However, with WFPB diet changes, people living with Type 1 diabetes can reduce their insulin needs and therefore their risk of complications while increasing their potential lifespan. This is crucial to know. Many Type 1 diabetics are told to simply adjust their insulin levels to what they eat, without being told that what they eat and when they eat are really important for improving the quality and length of their life.

Type 2 diabetes

Type 2 diabetes is caused primarily by insulin resistance. Insulin resistance is also at the root of other conditions such as polycystic ovarian syndrome and reduced fertility, as well as gestational diabetes. It also plays a part in the development of chronic kidney disease, fatty liver disease and even Alzheimer's. Over time, many Type 2 diabetics find their tired pancreas is worn out from going into overdrive all the time, trying to make more insulin in response to high blood sugars, and eventually it will stop working properly. This is why diabetes often progresses over time, and why some people ultimately need insulin to help.

Most Type 2 diabetics do not end up needing insulin and can improve their glucose sensitivity or their pancreatic overload through dietary changes, or they can use medications to improve their blood sugar levels. I have seen in my own patients that when they decide to adopt a WFPB diet, many of my Type 2 diabetics can stop taking insulin, and can even stop their tablets in some cases, as their glucose sensitivity rises. It is a joy to see.

THE EFFECT OF A WFPB DIET ON DIABETES

Our genes and age put us at risk of developing Type 2 diabetes. The good news is that your lifestyle choices can have the biggest impact on whether you will develop Type 2 diabetes or not.

Research shows that the more plant-based foods you eat, the lower your risk of Type 2 diabetes. One team of researchers conducted a comprehensive review and meta-analysis of nine studies looking at the association between dietary patterns and the risk of developing Type 2 diabetes. These studies involved 307,099 participants, of which 23,544 had Type 2 diabetes. They concluded that the people who ate a predominantly WFPB diet reduced their risk of diabetes by 23 per cent, compared to those who adhered less strictly to these dietary patterns. They also noted that the risk was even lower for those people who kept to a fully WFPB diet. They noted that these diets improve both insulin sensitivity and blood pressure, which both play a role in the development of diabetes. This way of eating also reduces weight gain and chronic low-grade inflammation, other factors that may lead to the development of diabetes.

WHY DOES INSULIN RESISTANCE HAPPEN?

This part is important to understand, and many doctors were not taught this physiology. Once you have understood this section, you will truly understand why plant-based diets help diabetes. Never again will you be scared by a banana or a potato!

In order to understand this, it is helpful to know what happens when we eat different nutrients. When we eat fatty foods, they tend to enter the bloodstream first, before glucose does. So, when you eat a doughnut, the fat in it absorbs before the glucose does. Fat causes the stomach-emptying speed to slow down, and the fatty acids are then absorbed in the small intestine as small fat globules called chylomicrons. These are carried into the blood where they reach the muscles first, before glucose and proteins can get there. Then the liver takes up what fat wasn't used and recirculates these fats in the blood as lipoproteins. You might have heard of LDL and HDL in your cholesterol blood test panel. These are abbreviations for small and large lipoproteins. These fatty acids are cholesterol transporters, and this process gives fats two chances to be absorbed by your body – first as chylomicrons, then as lipoproteins. They are used for energy or stored inside the muscle or liver cells for later.

The problem is your muscles can't reject this fat, and neither can your liver. There is no lock and key, it is an open door. So, although the liver and muscle cells prefer to store glycogen over fat, they end up storing this fat in lipid droplets within them. This causes fatty liver and fatty muscles. This process reduces the number and activity of the insulin receptors on the surface of your cells. They already have enough energy, and don't want any more energy from glucose, thank you very much. It's a case of first come, first served. Within hours of a high-fat meal, the receptors for insulin on the cell surface reduce in quantity and quality. This causes the muscle and liver cells to reject insulin. This is 'insulin resistance'. This occurs in polycystic ovary syndrome, and can eventually cause Type 2 diabetes, sometimes many years after the process has begun.

Normally glucose (sugar) is supposed to go into the muscle cells to power them, and into the liver cells for energy and to be stored as glycogen. But remember that glucose cannot get there by itself, it needs insulin to 'give permission' for it to enter into the cells. The insulin has to open the door. When these tiny fat particles build up inside the muscle cells (intra-myocellular lipid), they disrupt the signalling for the insulin keys and prevent them from being able to attach to the receptors properly. The lock is jammed, the key doesn't fit and the glucose has nowhere to go.

The result? Glucose is stuck in the bloodstream, causing toxicity in the blood vessels and nerves. If you are insulin resistant and your cells are filled with fat, the sugars that you eat will make your blood sugar levels rise very high. This can happen to anyone at any age. The pancreas notices and does the only thing it can do: it makes more insulin keys.

But it doesn't matter how many keys you make if the lock is jammed. The glucose is still stuck. Then you are left with two problems – not only too much glucose, but too much insulin as well. This is Type 2 diabetes.

What happens when the muscle cells and the liver cells are full of fatty acids, and there are still a lot of fatty acids left over in the blood? They can enter your fat tissue (adipose tissue) too. Adipose tissue is all over your body, not just your stomach or thighs. It is designed to grow and shrink in response to feast and famine, to provide energy when food isn't available. It also protects the muscles and liver from having to take all the load from excess fat in our food. But these fat cells can't expand without limit. After a while these cells can burst open and spill fatty acids into the fluid surrounding the tissue. This cell debris gets into the bloodstream and the neighbouring cells notice – they release stress signals called cytokines, which stimulate special clean up cells called macrophages to munch away at the cellular debris. But this process triggers long-term inflammation and increased risk of other diseases such as cancer.

Lastly, what does excess fat do to the pancreas itself? It stresses the beta cells which make insulin. These amazing little cells only make up 1 per cent of our pancreas. They are precious because we stop making them by about age 20. Sadly, fatty acids cause 'beta cell lipotoxicity' and can cause programmed cell death, or 'apoptosis'. This is bad news for the remaining beta cells because they have to work even harder to make insulin, unless the body can respond to insulin once more. This is end stage Type 2 diabetes, which usually requires insulin injections.

Pancreatic cell death happens in different people at different rates – but the good news is it will slow down dramatically if we can regain insulin sensitivity again. Even when many of these cells have died, a change in diet towards more whole plant foods can mean the remaining cells can boost their efficiency and begin to work normally. With a WFPB diet, my patients who were relying on insulin for managing their Type 2 diabetes have been able to come off it quickly. Studies also show reduced insulin needs on a WFPB diet even when bodyweight remains unchanged. It is truly incredible how quickly the body can adjust; within a matter of days your pancreas will be able to wake up and begin working once more.

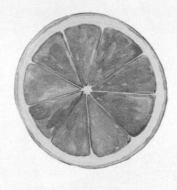
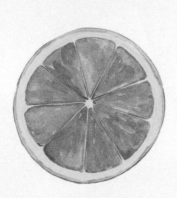

DIABETES – WHAT IS THE TRUTH ABOUT CARBS AND FIBRE?

People with diabetes are often told to cut the carbs because carbs break down into sugar, and sugar is 'bad' for diabetes. The truth is that carbs are a major food group and consist of sugars, starches and fibre-rich foods. So, although doughnuts are carbs, they are really refined sugar with fat mixed in. Fruit, vegetables, pulses, wholegrains and beans are all carbohydrate foods too, but they can provide not only glucose, which provides energy to the body and is the fuel that your brain prefers, but also fibre and nutrients that your body can use for other things.

Fibre has the ability to regulate blood sugar and even small increases in soluble fibre have been proven to help lower blood glucose levels. Eating fibre with our sugars slows down their rate of digestion and absorption by the body. This is why our blood sugars will spike after a glass of orange juice but will rise slowly when we eat an orange with all the extra stringy fibrous pith separating each segment. It also takes a lot longer to eat. Amazingly, fibre from legumes also causes something called 'the second meal effect' which means not only does it reduce the sugar response of the meal we are eating right now, but that of the next meal we eat, and even the one after that. This effect has been observed with lentils, chickpeas and beans. If you eat beans or lentils, you'll get less than half the insulin spike you'd get with the same amount of carbohydrates from pasta or potatoes. Why? It's the amazing short-chain fatty acids produced when our gut bugs break down fibre. Proprionate (one of the SCFAs) produced by good gut bugs when we eat beans, slows the rate at which food leaves our stomachs so we get less of a sugar rush.

This is one of the reasons why increasing the amount of fibre in your diet can help to manage diabetes. One study tested the effect two different meals had on blood sugar levels after eating; one dish was rice and the other, rice and beans. Seventeen participants who had Type 2 diabetes ate either white rice, white rice with kidney beans, white rice with black beans, or white rice with pinto beans. Their blood sugar was measured after 90 minutes and then again after two hours and two and a half hours. Compared with the men and women who ate just rice, all the groups that ate beans with rice had better blood sugar control. The participants who ate black beans and pinto beans saw the best results.

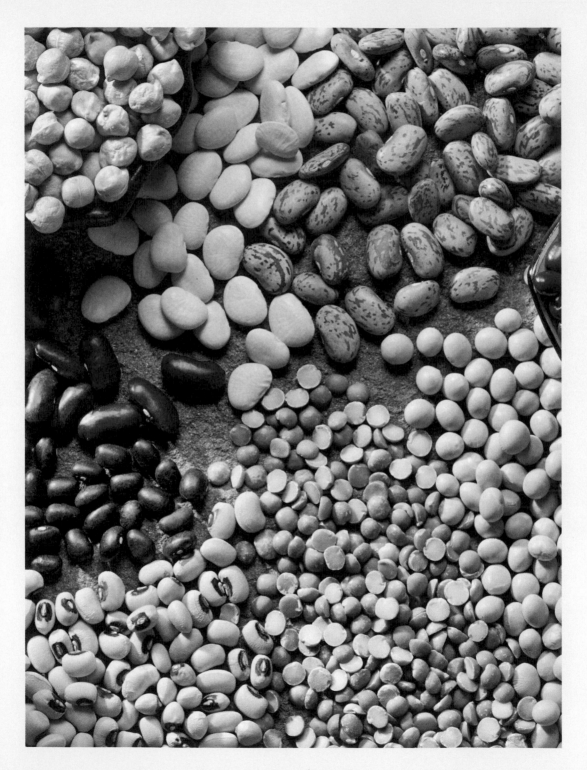

THE PLANT POWER DOCTOR

So you can see we need carbohydrates for longer, healthier lives. Many people try low-carb diets for weight loss and for diabetes control – and short-term studies show this can work primarily because of calorie restriction. You're eating less and cutting the amount of sugar in the bloodstream that the body has to deal with. The loss of the sugar spike means that less insulin is produced. As losing weight and reducing insulin levels are both helpful, people are then happy that their diabetes blood tests are looking better too, which reinforces this way of eating.

But be warned, this is not a long-term strategy for health. Glucose is a bit like petrol for the body. A low-carb diet is a like a rag in the petrol tank stopping you from putting in fuel – the car will run well for a while, but you can eventually drive into problems.

Carbohydrates are usually half or more of the average person's diet, if you take out not just the unhealthy snacks but foods such as rice, fruit, beans, pasta and bread, chances are you will lose weight as a net effect of reducing caloric intake. If you make up for it with meat and cheese, you won't necessarily lose any weight. Studies show that the low-carb eaters who tend to lose weight are the ones who reduce their overall intake of calories. More worrisome is what happens in the blood. Remember how saturated fat clogs up the insulin receptors? If you eat a steak, it's the fat in the steak clogging up the receptors, which then means your body can't process that healthy apple you tried to eat afterwards.

Another concern about high-fat, low-carb diets is your blood cholesterol levels. If you lose weight, however you do it, typically your cholesterol will drop too. But this doesn't always happen when on a low-carb diet, where a significant minority of people eating this way can actually have a rise in their lipid profiles despite weight loss. A study published in 2012 also showed that a low-carbohydrate, high-protein and high-fat diet stiffened peripheral arteries, which made the small blood vessels less responsive, and less able to swell and constrict. This increases the risk of high blood pressure, heart attacks and stroke.

Similarly, a study directly comparing the heart arteries of patients on a healthy low-carb diet vs a healthy high-carb diet showed significantly reduced blood flow to the heart (the coronary arteries) with the low-carb diet. Long term, this means potential for increased risk of premature death in low-carb dieters who focus on animal sources of protein over plant proteins.

So, my advice is that although low-carb diets can be beneficial for controlling blood sugars or weight loss, they are not an optimally healthy long-term solution. If you have benefited from a low-carb approach in the past and you have good results, that's great. But armed with this information, you have the option of a different choice. For your long-term health, and for sustainability. After all, we would need eight planet Earths if we all ate an animal-based keto diet.

At the end of this chapter there are some actionable points so you can reduce your risk of developing diabetes or maybe even stop it in its tracks.

CAN A WFPB DIET REVERSE DIABETES?

Generally healthy lifestyles with good sleep, stress reduction, meditation and exercise are all very beneficial. But what has the potential to dramatically improve – or even reverse – Type 2 diabetes long term?

My first clue in answering this question came from a patient I was treating some years ago. He was a charismatic man, but life had dealt him difficult cards. Despite being in his early forties, he had severe heart disease and diabetes. He had already suffered a heart attack and had very raised cholesterol levels. He also had complications from his diabetes including impotence and neuropathy (nerve pains). But despite his medical woes, he took a trip to the Caribbean. While there, he was locked up in prison for drug-smuggling – not a man for a quiet life, it seems!

But here's the thing. While he was in prison, what was he fed each day? Rice and beans. The ultimate high-carb diet. What happened? His diabetes improved dramatically. He was able to come off his medications and he was in the best shape of his life. This greatly confused me, as much of what I understood at that time was around carbs being 'bad' for diabetes. On his return home, I was amazed at his improvements. But his eating habits did not return with him, and sadly his improvements did not last either. Back to the bacon and eggs, and his diabetes returned with a vengeance.

What became clear with my patient, and of course when I understood the mechanisms of insulin resistance, was that the optimal eating pattern to lessen the effects of diabetes – or even reverse the diagnosis – is a WFPB-lifestyle approach. Replacing foods rich in saturated fat with carbohydrate-rich wholefoods will dissipate the fat inside the cells, allowing the insulin key to work again and let glucose into the cell where it is needed for energy. Replacing saturated fats with polyunsaturated fats (PUFAs) from foods like nuts, seeds, avocados and olives will also improve insulin sensitivity to a point – but remember a little goes a long way. Potatoes, sweetcorn, mangoes, squash, beans, lentils, quinoa and bananas can all come back on the menu. It usually only takes a matter of days for your pancreas to wake up, your cell receptors to work again and for your glucose sensitivity to rise.

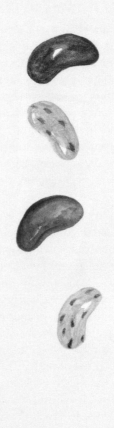

This should be done with careful monitoring of your blood sugars if you are on tablets or insulin because it is likely to cause a dramatic drop in circulating blood sugar. This shows your cells are becoming more responsive to insulin again, and that the changes are working. It will be important to see your doctor to talk about reducing your oral medications if you are on them and reduce your insulin requirements too. Doctors will be unfamiliar with the speed with which insulin sensitivity can rise, and so you must be aware that serious hypos can occur if you are on certain tablets or insulin without monitoring. Amazingly, with these dietary changes, it is possible to reverse some of these conditions and take back control of your health.

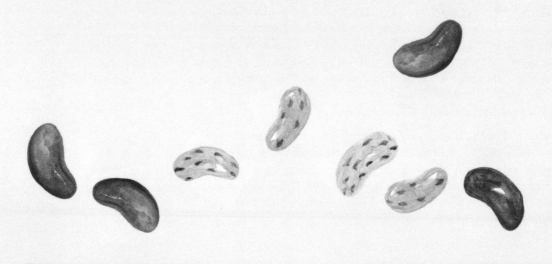

TWO OTHER WAYS TO INCREASE INSULIN SENSITIVITY

The quality and quantity of the foods you eat are two of the most important predictors of your metabolic health when you are living with diabetes. How do we measure metabolic health? Checking blood sugar control, blood pressure, lipid profile and waist circumference to name a few; these are all markers that doctors use to calculate the risk of developing chronic diseases like diabetes and heart disease. They help us decide if the patient in front of us is 'metabolically healthy'. Food, movement, sleep and stress all play a part in improving or jeopardising our metabolic health. Let's take a closer look at ways – other than food – to increase insulin sensitivity and thereby improve metabolic health.

Fasting

Changing the timing of your food intake has been shown to be particularly effective for improving insulin sensitivity. It can free stored fat – including the fat stored within your muscles and liver – which means the pancreas can work more efficiently. For thousands of years, we were largely 'gatherer-hunters' and due to food scarcity at certain times and places, we had to adapt to periods of fasting and be able to survive. Scientists in the 1930s observed that mice who were forced to restrict their food intake lived longer than those who could eat whenever they wanted. This observation triggered an explosion of research trying to understand the biological mechanisms that result in boosted longevity, memory and weight loss, and reduced risk of chronic diseases such as diabetes, cancer and dementia. The same kind of pathways seem to exist in all organisms studied – from yeast to flies and from monkeys to humans. However, in the real world, calorie restriction can be hugely challenging – and will not suit everyone. We have yet to fully understand how fasting affects the resilience of our gut bug populations, for better or for worse. If you are someone who has had problems with disordered eating, such as bulimia or anorexia, or feeling unable to eat unless you have exercised, my clinical experience would suggest that fasting will not suit you.

If you do want to give intermittent fasting a try, there are many types of fasting regimes to choose from, so which one is best? There are several options, including alternate-day fasting, daily caloric restriction (about 25 per cent fewer calories each day) or a once a week fast (for 24 hours). The list is not exhaustive, but I feel the choices below are the easiest.

- **The 16:8 daily fast:** Eat within an 8-hour window every day.

- **The 5-day Fasting Mimicking Diet:** Consume 500–600 calories every day for five days from soups, herbal teas and healthy snacks. This can be done once every six months or so.

- **The 5:2 regime:** Eat reduced calories two days a week of between 500 to 600 calories. The other days eat as you normally would.

Needless to say, if you are an insulin-dependent diabetic you will need to consult with a doctor or dietician before trying this in order to modify your medication schedule while fasting. Never fast for more than three days without medical supervision. If you have poor glycogen stores and suffer rapid mood swings or shakes while attempting a true fast, a modified fast may be better. That is, having 100–200-calorie snacks instead of avoiding food entirely. Other top tips include drinking lots of water and herbal teas – especially green tea which is quite useful for curbing the appetite. If you don't think fasting is for you, the good news is that you can still get results by simply switching to a wholefoods plant-based approach.

Exercise

Movement is good for mitochondria, the small structures in our cells that are like batteries and power them. Over the last few years, studies have shown that people with Type 2 diabetes tend to have less mitochondria in their muscle cells, and those they do have can be less efficient. Exercise allows your muscles to make more – by contracting those muscle fibres you stimulate mitochondria that are needed to process more oxygen the next time muscles are required to move. Exercise can also substitute insulin to a degree – this is because muscle contractions force the muscles to use up their glycogen and triglyceride stores and burn glucose and fatty acids at the same time. Glucose is preferred for short bursts and fatty acids for longer duration exercise. How can you optimise insulin sensitivity and burn more fatty acids? Combining 'short of breath' exercise and resistance exercise is great, and three hours a week of exercise spread out over six or seven days will be better for keeping your insulin sensitivity higher at all times.

If you inject insulin, you will need to experiment to find a regime that suits your insulin needs – elevating blood glucose beforehand to prevent hypos can be a strategy, which can be done by reducing your pre-workout insulin dose or by eating a small breakfast and injecting 30–60 minutes before exercise. This is a process of trial and error.

The main takeaway here is that any form of exercise is better than nothing. The best regime is one that you can fit into your day consistently. And that although these strategies for intermittent fasting and exercising are really useful, we simply can't out-exercise a poor diet. The quality of the foods you eat is the most important indicator of long-term metabolic health when you are living with diabetes.

TOP TIPS FOR DIABETES PREVENTION AND REVERSAL

Find your 'why': If you have your goals, desires and new identity at the forefront of your mind, these changes become much easier.

Keep a food diary: Consider keeping a food log for two days before you make changes so you can be aware of what you are changing in advance.

Eat more wholefoods and plants: This should include fruit, starchy veg, legumes, greens, mushrooms, herbs and spices.

Eat fewer high-fat and high-sugar foods: Cut out or reduce your intake of meat, eggs, dairy, oil and processed junk foods.

Daily flax seeds: This will help you reach your omega-3 fatty acid goals.

Exercise regularly.

Introduce time-restricted eating: This will allow for improved weight regulation and insulin sensitivity.

Get enough B12 and vitamin D: Take a supplement or get your vitamin D from sunlight.

Reduce your stress.

Regulate your sleep.

Share your success: If you are on insulin or medications, it is be crucial to seek the support and guidance of your doctor to help you reduce your medications safely.

CASE STUDY – CYRUS'S STORY

Cyrus is not a patient of mine but a friend who has written about living with Type 1 diabetes. Cyrus was diagnosed with Type 1 diabetes when he was 22 and studying at Stanford University. His diagnosis came on top of two previous diagnoses within the previous six months. At that time, he had also developed two other autoimmune conditions, making diabetes his third autoimmune condition. His doctors diagnosed polyglandular autoimmune syndrome, a term used to describe a collection of autoimmune conditions with no known cause. His doctors had never seen this before and, aged just 22, he was terrified that his health was failing, even though he led a healthy lifestyle.

He did his best to remain calm and practical, but Cyrus felt lonely and scared. He found controlling his blood glucose more difficult than he had anticipated. The literature he read consistently told him to follow a low-carb diet but as hard as he tried, he struggled to keep his glucose within a 'normal' range.

He said, 'I felt out of shape, excessively tired and downright confused – I was a 22-year-old living in what felt like the body of a 90-year-old. No matter how hard I tried, no matter how many variables I worked to control, no matter how systematic I was at documenting my daily activities, my blood glucose monitor acted like a random number generator, which frustrated me beyond belief.'

Cyrus decided to take matters into his own hands and began to experiment. He searched high and low for information and found that much of his research pointed him towards plant-based eating. Eventually he turned to biochemistry and worked with a nutritionist and began eating a WFPB diet.

He said: 'In the first week of eating a strictly plant-based diet, my insulin requirements dropped by around 35 per cent, my energy levels increased, and my blood glucose became significantly more predictable. I calculated that my carbohydrate intake had increased almost sixfold, from about 75 grams per day to about 500 grams per day. That means that I was eating significantly more carbohydrate and using less insulin, which went against everything that I had been told since day one. This made no sense at all. When I began eating more carbohydrate-rich foods, I found that my biological requirement for insulin dropped significantly and quickly.'

This personal account correlates with the scientific data, and if Cyrus's story sounds familiar, it could be that for you too, restricting carbohydrates may be harming rather than helping your body.

RESET YOUR SKIN

They say the eyes are the window to the soul. If that's true, our skin is the bricks and mortar. Our skin is a truly incredible organ that does so much for us, and it can be devastatingly evident when the skin starts to go wrong. It is the largest organ in the body, providing us with an important barrier to the outside world and regulating many systems in the body, such as our temperature, vitamin D production and wound healing. Skin should be treated with care, and one of the best ways to do that is by providing it with the right hydration and nutrients.

Many people only start focusing on the skin when there is a problem. Sometimes the cell turnover process or the protective barrier can break down and not only can this cause physical pain, but it can be emotionally challenging as the perception of our skin is interwoven with feelings of wellness, vitality and youth. Other people's opinions of how we look can also make us feel bad when our skin is affected by medical conditions such as acne, eczema or psoriasis. Because we can see the skin, it is usually very obvious when something is going wrong. However, what is not so obvious is the diagnosis, or the underlying causes of these problems.

Diet and skin health are closely linked, and by eating healthy foods you can also nourish your skin from the inside out. Medical interventions are often really important too, and seeing a doctor early if your skin is in trouble will be helpful in deciding your diagnosis and what treatments to try.

Why not also try other lifestyle changes to help your skin at the same time? With a WFPB diet you will be eating more nutrient-rich foods, including the building blocks of vitamins A, C, E and other antioxidants, which work hard to keep your skin healthy. It is important to note that it can be a long road, with bumps and detours along the way.

Instead of eating without thinking about the effect it could have on our skin, let's nourish it as we would every other organ, and give it some love and attention from the inside out.

ACNE

If you suffer from acne and it is affecting your mood, don't suffer in silence because the psychological effects can be devastating. My mother had severe cystic acne when I was growing up, and I saw first hand how it changed her personality and self-confidence. I myself have struggled and can have bad days when I have not taken care of my diet, or my stress, or my skincare routine. It is not trivial, and teenagers should not be told 'you'll grow out of it'. I have seen so many teenagers whose views of the world and how they fit into it have been shaped by acne.

Many of us in the Western world can suffer acne at any time in our lives. Acne develops when dead skin cells and your skin's natural oils block the hair follicles in your skin. Bacteria enter the blocked follicles and start multiplying. When your immune blood cells try to defend themselves against the bacteria, this can cause redness, swelling and spots.

Acne affects up to 85 per cent of teenagers in the Western world as hormones like testosterone and oestrogen affect how much sebum is produced and how oily the skin becomes, but for many of us it also persists into adulthood. Yet, some cultures do not have issues with acne at all.

For many years, we were told that diet had very little to do with acne, that it was stress, genetics and hormones – and bad luck. More research is now establishing specific enzyme pathways that can lead to acne in susceptible people – and that diet can indeed improve this for some of us. Others will have a very healthy diet and still suffer, and there is no magic formula. We will come on to the other causes in a moment, but first let's deal with what's easy to shift: food choices.

Dairy, junk foods, meat, and egg proteins in Western diets all have an impact on a specific enzyme pathway in the body known as TOR which acts to drive cellular growth and metabolic processes (see page 34). Overstimulation of this TOR enzyme pathway can contribute to premature puberty as well as acne. This means that milk, cheese and butter are not just foods, but they are also signals to the body, causing overstimulation of this important process. Why is this overstimulation a potential problem? Because cow's milk is designed for calves. Cow infants grow nearly 40 times faster than human infants. Cow's milk has three times more leucine (an amino

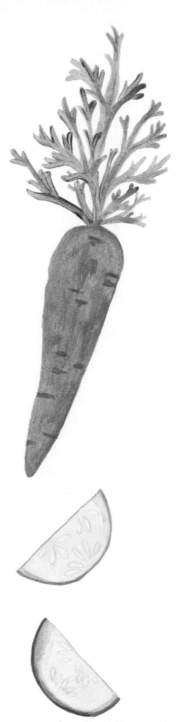

acid) than human milk, which is one of the primary activators of TOR. Leucine also increases cellular ageing, according to the Nobel-prize-nominated research of Professor Valter Longo along with that of many other longevity researchers. Leucine, and all essential amino acids, are crucial in the right amounts, and can be found in foods such as beans, peanut butter, tofu and seeds. But it is about creating a balance. Our foods should provide us with enough valuable nutrients and amino acids – but we can sometimes get too much of a good thing.

Eating more fruits and vegetables, wholegrains and legumes will reduce these effects. Plant foods are packed with antioxidants, nutrients and fibre to improve your skin. Oranges and lemons contain vitamin C, tomatoes contain lycopene, sweet potatoes are rich in beta-carotene (to make vitamin A), leafy greens and yellow vegetables contain lutein, and nuts, seeds, spinach and avocado contain vitamin E – all these vitamins help maintain skin health so the bigger the variety of plant foods the better!

Late nights, alcohol, coffee, junk food, lack of sleep or anabolic steroids for muscle building – all these things can potentially have an effect on spots. Sweating from exercise, saunas and especially outdoor activity is ideal for keeping the biome healthy because sweat supports the healthy balance of skin bacteria. But leaving sweaty clothes on all day should be avoided if you can! Aim to make your daily habits as restorative as possible. We all have off days – just notice them so you can get back on track if you need to.

SUGAR, GREASE AND GLUTEN

Bad news for chocolate lovers. Refined sugar can cause inflammation in the body, and chocolate is the worst culprit when it comes to spots, it seems. Especially white chocolate, which is high in sugar and fat, but even dark chocolate and cocoa powder can be problematic. Cocoa seems to be linked to acne outbreaks – even in a blind placebo-controlled trial where people were given cocoa powder in capsule form. So, it's wise to limit chocolate for a while if you suffer from acne.

Greasy foods have been shown to increase sebum production, which can contribute to breakouts. So, avoiding pastries, pies and cakes as much as possible is good advice. Increasing the omega-3 fatty acid ratio in the diet may help reduce the risk. Increasing consumption of flax seeds, chia seeds and walnuts over other healthy fats is a good way forward. Algae supplements such as EPA/DHA contain the purest form of long chain omega-3 fatty acids, which may be useful if you avoid fish. This may also benefit your skin.

What about gluten-free diets? For most of us, gluten is not an issue when it comes to skin health – especially if we have a healthy microbiome. However, it is still important to stick to wholegrains over refined grains. For those who are gluten sensitive, a gluten elimination trial may help. This is a trial and error approach. If you decide to eliminate gluten, and you notice no difference after a few weeks, it is highly unlikely that you would have an issue with grains. Gluten-free diets are only useful for people with coeliac disease or perhaps non-coeliac gluten sensitivity. Wholegrains on the other hand have been shown in many studies to be associated with good health and longevity, so it is worth including them unless you have a specific reason not to. It is also worth noting that some forms of gluten may be more digestible than others, e.g. spelt rather than wholewheat. People who are sensitive can focus on the abundance of wholegrains and pseudo-grains that are naturally gluten-free such as oats, red rice, quinoa, amaranth and buckwheat.

ECZEMA

Eczema presents as itchy, inflamed, swollen and crusty patches of skin. It is thought to have an immune component, and the underlying changes in the body are very similar with atopic (usually inherited) eczema, asthma and hay fever. All are due to allergic reactions where the immune system reacts to normally harmless substances. They are all classed as 'type 1 hypersensitivity'. Our immune system has millions of antibodies and each one recognises a specific invader. In people with allergies, antibodies called IgE are formed when someone is exposed to a 'harmless' invader or allergen such as pollen, cat or dog saliva, feathers, cow's milk, eggs, shellfish, etc.

These antibodies attach to mast cells which are present in large numbers in the mucous lining of the respiratory and digestive tracts and in skin tissue. On re-exposure to the allergen, the IgE antibody grabs hold of it and tells the mast cell to release chemicals, which provoke an allergic response.

You may have heard of the main chemical that causes inflammation – histamine. This is why 'anti-histamines' are given to dampen down allergic inflammation, such as with hay fever or itchy eczema. Inflammation is normally a good thing if you are fighting a harmful invader, but in the case of eczema, asthma and hay fever, it is an over-reaction to a harmless substance. Inflammation means that blood capillaries widen allowing more blood to flow to the area, bringing more antibodies to fight the invader. The increased blood flow causes redness and warmth. Water also seeps from the capillaries in an attempt to dilute any poisons that may be at the site – this causes swelling. If the mast cells 'switched on' by the IgE antibodies are located in the mucous lining of the nose, they also cause the production of excessive mucous and so a runny nose is the result. If the mast cells are in the lining of the lungs, the histamine and other chemicals also cause contraction of, and mucous production in, the airways, leading to blockage or asthma. If the allergic response happens in the skin, then it's labelled eczema.

The tendency is for all three conditions to run in families, and yet if an identical twin has eczema, in one-in-five cases the other twin will not develop symptoms. This is because all allergies have triggers that differ from person to person. You can potentially switch some of these hereditary triggers off through improving gut health and eating a more plant-focused diet.

WHAT CAUSES ECZEMA?

Irritants like soap, detergent and bubble bath as well as cold or dry weather can be triggers. As for causes, I suspect the gut microbiome plays an enormous role in which allergies occur, and also helps to dictate which genes are switched on and off in each individual. The acid mantle of our epidermis that develops at birth has an important barrier function, as well as maintaining a microbiome environment on the skin to prevent eczema. The skin barrier can be negatively affected by certain things beyond our control, such as Caesarean section delivery, antibiotics exposures, or not being breastfed. In adults, diet, hormones, environmental triggers and stress can all play a part in the development and the severity of eczema.

In children, one of the main triggers is food – cow's milk, eggs and nuts are the top three contributors. Others in the top seven are house dust mites, fish, soya and wheat. It's also worth being aware that if a child has eczema and a nut allergy, they are 80 per cent more likely to develop asthma later in childhood. Adults with eczema may be more likely to react to birch pollen-associated foods like apples, carrots, celery and hazelnuts.

Another trigger is infection – infected areas of already vulnerable or broken skin are a big component of eczema. Many people with eczema are nasal carriers of a bacteria called staphylococcus aureus. All they have to do is rub their nose or sneeze and then scratch their skin and they can develop a secondary infection overnight. Staph aureus also reduces the amount of steroid receptors on the skin, which means steroid creams have to be stronger to have an effect. If you a prone to infected eczema, the good news is that dealing with infections early using a nasal antibiotic, and swabbing the nose if necessary, can be useful in getting things under control.

The third trigger for flare-ups is stress. Breathing techniques, mindfulness, meditation, exercise, building social networks, me-time and many other self-care practices can help with this. Being aware of stress as a trigger can encourage you to look for solutions that are not just focused on the skin.

TREATMENTS

Moisturisers are an important component of treatment, providing relief of itching and pain. Steroids are used by doctors for flare-ups, whereas moisturisers are more of a basic treatment. They don't penetrate into the deeper layers of skin – but are useful for symptom control and prevention. Severe cases will be seen by a dermatologist for other treatments targeting the immune system, and they may also use light therapies.

Skincare routines that include hyaluronic acid, antioxidants (vitamins A, C and E) and SPF are usually suggested by skin experts too. There is not enough data on this for me to advise whether probiotics are useful, but they are used a lot in the skin industry, so perhaps time will tell.

DIET AND ECZEMA

It's known that some foods trigger allergies, while others protect us. The most common foods linked to eczema are cow's milk (the number one culprit!) and eggs. Lesser triggers are fish, soya, wheat and nuts, according to the National Eczema Society.

Remember how eczema, asthma and hay fever are all related to each other? Some foods help protect against allergies more generally. For example, research has shown that people who ate the most fruit and vegetables had the healthiest lung function. Vitamin C (from fresh fruit and vegetables) and E (from nuts and seeds, avocados, tomatoes, wholegrains etc.) are also believed to help reduce the severity of the inflammatory response in the lungs of people with asthma. To provide another example of how diet affects allergies, studies have shown that if a breastfeeding mum's diet is high in animal fats and low in omega-3, the risk of her baby developing allergic conditions increases.

Limiting or avoiding processed foods has also shown to be of benefit in many children with eczema. I have seen this with my own patients, and parents have come back to me delighted when their son or daughter has improved, when all they changed was cutting out processed meat and sweets. One mum even said to me, 'Why has no doctor ever told me this before?' I didn't have a good answer for her. Especially in light of studies such as this one – the Korean National Health and Nutrition examination of over 17,000 people, which found that those whose diets contained the highest amounts of meats and processed foods had a 57 per cent greater risk for atopic dermatitis (eczema) when compared with individuals whose diets contained the least.

Additionally, the International Study on Asthma and Allergy in Children (ISAAC) performed in Colombia found that children whose diets contained the highest amounts of traditionally eaten foods, such as fresh fruit and legumes, had an almost 40 per cent lower risk of having eczema, compared to those eating the lowest amounts of these foods.

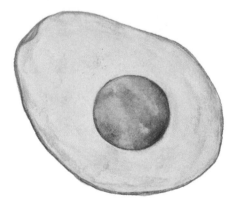

Allergies are now so common in the UK that the Royal College of Physicians is referring to them as an epidemic of the skin. Although there is a strong genetic component involved, it is essential to boost your health and improve the functioning of your immune system to minimise the chances of a flare-up. This means: eat a healthy diet rich in fruit, vegetables, nuts, seeds, wholegrains and omega-3s. Exercising regularly helps keep the heart, bones and digestive system healthy and keeps excess weight off. Find ways to make yourself feel good and better able to cope with the stresses of everyday life too.

CASE STUDY – JANE'S STORY

Jane had struggled with breakouts of acne for the last two years. It started on her shoulders, then on her back and chest. She was able to cover this up with clothes but then it started to affect her neck and face and was now visible for everyone to see. She had always looked after her skin and had an interest in skincare. She pared down her skincare regimen, removed any products that contained active ingredients or perfume to avoid skin irritation.

She eventually visited her GP (which was not me) who tried her on multiple antibiotics and peroxide cream yet after three months nothing was clearing her acne. They did refer her to see a dermatologist but due to Covid-19 that appointment was postponed indefinitely.

She then saw an ad for the Happy Pear skin course online, which is a four-week cooking programme with skincare education that I have had the pleasure in helping chefs David and Stephen Flynn to provide. After having no luck with any other skin treatments, she thought she had nothing to lose, so she signed up. She said that what really made a difference for her was a shift in food, and the focus on getting as much fresh fruit, vegetables and fibre as possible into each meal. There was no focus on restrictions or what she couldn't have.

She said the difference to her skin after four weeks was something she did not expect. Her skin is clearer and much brighter now and while she still has the occasional flare-up, it's much milder and perhaps only noticeable to her. She puts this down to the power of plants.

HORMONES AND HEALTH

Hormones play an integral role in our health. Incredibly, there are more than 50 hormones within us and they affect every part of our lives, including growth, metabolism, appetite, puberty and fertility. We can think of our hormones in terms of an orchestra. If you imagine every individual musician and instrument playing perfectly in tune and the conductor (the brain) is doing his job well, then all the hormones come in at the right place and work in the right way. You will have a beautiful symphony. If the conductor is off, the violin is screechy or the bassist is having a bad day, it will become a cacophony of noise. And even the smallest imbalance can set this off. Factors that affect our hormones include everything from what we put on our skin and the things we eat and breathe, to different lifestyle factors, such as getting enough exercise and sleep.

HOW DO HORMONES WORK?

Hormones are the chemical messengers in our bodies. They are usually made by glands, which operate in an amazing feedback loop with other glands to regulate all the body's functions. Glands are all part of the endocrine system.

The testes or ovaries are perhaps the most familiar of these endocrine glands. In males, testes produce sperm and secrete the male sex hormone testosterone and in females, ovaries produce eggs and release oestrogen. These hormones therefore play a role in sperm production, periods and pregnancy. Other important glands include the thyroid and adrenal glands. Hormones can only affect cells that have receptors that are specific to them, but some cells will have receptors to many different hormones at the same time. For example, the hormone that the thyroid produces acts on many different tissues, which is why its effects are so wide-ranging. The same with insulin, which can act on many different types of cell and is known as the body's best 'transporter hormone'.

Haywire hormones can affect everyone at every stage of life; and ageing means that we produce more of certain hormones and less of others. For example, in women the most obvious example of hormonal changes is the menopause, where women's ovaries produce decreasing amounts of oestrogen and progesterone. So many of my patients struggle with awful symptoms at this stage in life, which is something we have to talk more about both within the medical profession and in the wider world. When hormones are crashing it can feel completely overwhelming, leading not only to flushing and sweats but also low mood, anxiety and even thoughts of suicide.

WHAT ARE HORMONE IMBALANCES?

Hormone imbalances are when there is too much or too little of a hormone in the bloodstream. Common hormonal symptoms that affect both men and women can include weight gain, mood swings, insomnia, fatigue, dry skin, low libido, muscle weakness, depression and skin problems. Women may experience heavy or irregular periods, fibroids and night sweats, whereas men may suffer from erectile dysfunction, acne, development of breast tissue or loss of muscle mass. These are just a handful of examples; hormone imbalances may be to blame for a host of unwanted symptoms.

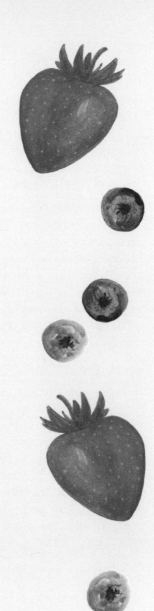

What can we do to get the orchestra playing in tune? Many things, including medications, minimising stress, exercising regularly, maintaining a healthy weight, getting enough sleep and cutting back on alcohol. But funnily enough, food can also play a starring role in your hormonal orchestra too. Without the right nutrients, our body struggles to make the correct hormones in the right amounts for optimal health. Western diets, lacking in whole, nutrient-dense foods, miss out the vital building blocks we need for keeping our hormones in check. But the great thing is, it doesn't have to be this way. I am going to go through some of the major conditions in our lives that can be mediated by hormones and, crucially, how you can start to take back control of this delightful symphony and create hormonal balance.

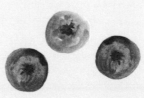

THE IMPORTANCE OF 'GOOD' FATS FOR HORMONES

Fat can have a bad reputation, and there is a lot of confusion on this topic. So, let's clarify a few things. Fat is one of the most important nutrients for hormone balance because healthy fats are essential for hormone production and the maintenance of proper hormone function. Our bodies use cholesterol as a backbone for all the hormones we make, and omega-3 fatty acids are anti-inflammatory and modulate hormone receptor site sensitivity.

That's why when people talk about 'low-fat diets' they are really describing the ideal situation of minimising excess fats from processed foods, junk food, processed oils and excess animal products, not eliminating fats altogether. Fats also help with the absorption of some vitamins, including vitamins A, D, E and K. So, enjoying a palmful of unsalted mixed nuts and a variety of seeds, as well as other healthy fats like avocados and olives will enhance your hormonal health and keep that symphony playing all the right notes.

WOMEN AND HORMONES

Women – I'm talking to you. And men, if you're reading this part your sisters, wives, mothers, daughters and friends will be glad that you did – so stick with me. From the moment when we first experience that distinctive cramping lower tummy pain, that dragging in the legs and sore breasts, we had a very real understanding of how tough hormones can be. Period pains, heavy bleeding each month, and conditions intimately linked with hormones – such as pre-menstrual stress, fibroids, endometriosis, polycystic ovaries, pregnancy and, of course, menopause – all serve to remind us that the quality of our lives are dictated by these hormones and how they affect us, from the age of ten or eleven onwards.

Let's start with periods. Interestingly, as the years go by, periods seem to be starting younger. Why is that? We have more access to food, and are growing taller too, so it stands to reason that earlier periods are just another part of this healthy trend, right? Not necessarily. When periods begin, bone growth is essentially done. Premature puberty is a serious problem because it is linked to greater risk of breast cancer, heart disease, diabetes and even adult-onset asthma. The high-fat, low-fibre Western diet, as well

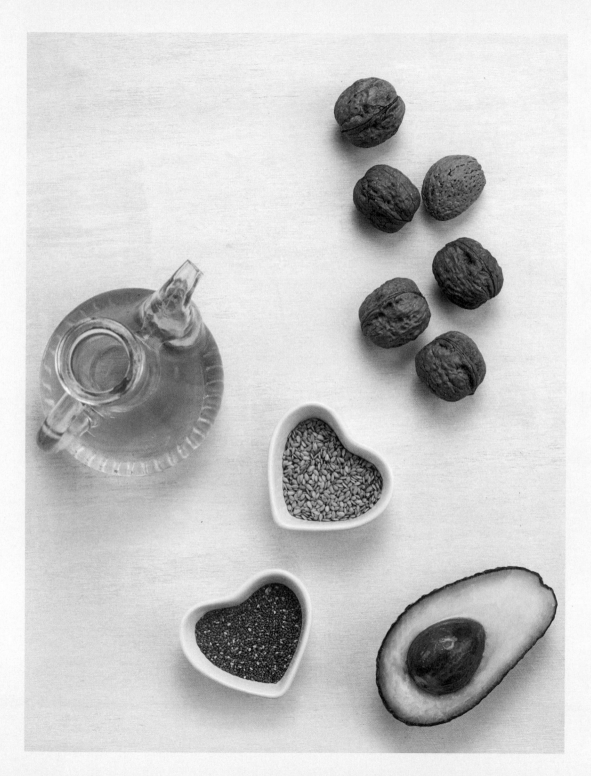

as reduced exercise, advances the onset of puberty for our young women, who may not be ready psychologically for the onset of womanhood, let alone the physical aspects of it. Women in the Western world also tend to go through menopause later, which means our lifetime exposure to oestrogen is higher, and puts us at increased risk of hormone-dependent cancers. What can we do? It's all about getting the right balance. We need oestrogen, but just not in excess.

Maintaining a normal weight, moving our bodies and making sure we visit the toilet regularly are a great start because being overweight can in itself mean we have a higher hormone exposure. This is because our fat cells are not just globules of lipid but are actually mini-hormone factories. They can make oestrogen and testosterone. This is why polycystic ovaries are linked to being overweight, and another reason why our weight plays a part in our lifetime cancer risk.

Being constipated is another way of being over-exposed to oestrogen. This is because the body discards excess hormones and products of metabolism through our poop. When we get bunged up, those waste products seep back into our bodies through the intestinal wall and get re-metabolised. This increases our hormonal exposure. In helping us make large soft stools, a high-fibre diet can be useful for hormonal regulation.

Pollutants are also a serious problem for our hormonal orchestra. Plastics and insecticides can have hormone-mimicking effects and have been linked to breast and prostate cancer. In fact, as an example, many studies on phthalates (chemicals used to help the durability and flexibility of plastics) shows they disrupt our hormones and have been linked to developmental issues, fertility problems and obesity. One study shows us a mechanism by which phthalates induce proliferation and invasiveness of breast cancers.

PERIOD PAINS

What happens in a woman's monthly cycles? Put simply, oestrogen levels are lowest just before and during our monthly period. The ovaries then release oestrogen to reach a peak two weeks later, which stimulates ovulation. Then oestrogen dips a little and gradually rises again to thicken up the womb lining ready for a pregnancy. If the egg is not fertilised, oestrogen falls rapidly and the thickened lining of the womb is lost in the monthly period blood.

As the lining breaks down, prostaglandins are released by womb-lining (endometrial) cells, which constrict blood vessels, cause womb contraction, induce pain and increase bleeding. They can also cause nausea, vomiting and diarrhoea if they enter the bloodstream. So, if there is too much oestrogen, what happens? The womb lining builds up more than it should. And if there are too many prostaglandins, the cramping and pain is also worse. This is why oral contraceptives help; they inhibit prostaglandins by reducing the growth of these womb lining cells. Anti-inflammatory painkillers can help too by reducing the production of prostaglandins. And here is where food can also play its part.

By eating foods rich in wholegrains and fibre, women can reduce the amount of excess oestrogen cycling within our bodies, and hopefully can also reduce the size of our fat cells. By eating less foods that stimulate prostaglandins, such as omega-6 fatty acids in vegetable oils, fatty foods and processed meat and dairy, we may also see a benefit. One crossover study showed this trend very well. Two months of a healthy WFPB diet reduced the intensity of period pain, and the duration of pain too. The researchers also found increased sex-hormone-binding globulin (SHBG) in the bloodstream. SHBG is an important protein molecule that holds onto hormones, storing them until they are needed, like a parachute backpack. Once the hormone is needed, the SHBG releases it and the parachute can open up and facilitate safe landing. For context, women who are overweight and who suffer with polycystic ovaries tend to have lower SHBG, which means they have more active hormones. In this way, SHBG has a really important role in regulating hormone expression.

The other interesting thing about this study was that the women also reported increased energy, better digestion and better sleep. When the women who were in the food group were required to ditch their plant-based diet to switch over to the placebo pill supplement group, many women refused, despite the conditions of the study. They wanted to stick with a way of eating that had helped them so much.

What else might help period pains? Vitamin D. There are vitamin D receptors in the womb and one trial showed us that with a single high-dose vitamin D treatment period pains could potentially be reduced. This is thought to be because vitamin D reduces prostaglandins. Ginger has been shown in another study to be equally as effective as two different types of anti-inflammatory

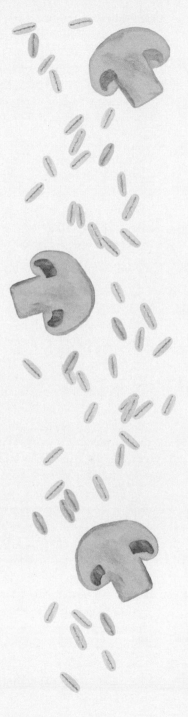

painkiller. Curcumin from turmeric has also been shown to have a potential benefit – the polyphenols are thought to increase BDNF levels (brain derived neurotropic factor) which improves period pains but is also known to help neurons survive and grow. A trial used two curcumin capsules daily from seven days before the period compared with a placebo pill. The women did this for three cycles and found improved mood, reduced pain and increased BDNF levels.

So, what can you do if you suffer from period pains? Why not aim to eat lots of fibre-rich plant foods throughout the month, take in good amounts of turmeric and ginger just before your period starts and throughout, as well as adding a vitamin D supplement if your levels are low? You may notice some big improvements within a few cycles and it could be an easy win to fit into your daily routine.

A WORD ABOUT THE PILL

The oral contraceptive pill has been a lifeline for many women over the years to externally regulate their cycle and minimise the effects of period pain. Combined oral contraceptives (COCPs) temporarily suspend the normal symphony between the hypothalamus, pituitary and ovaries by drafting in an external band of players – a pill containing external oestrogen and progesterone. This can improve period pains a lot, especially if taken back to back for women with heavy periods or endometriosis. It also has the bonus of providing a reliable contraceptive, which can reduce the risk of ovarian, uterine and colorectal cancers. There are other effects too though – it can increase the risk of elevated blood pressure, migraines, gallstones, reduced libido, blood clotting (particularly if a woman is over 35 years old, a smoker, overweight or hypertensive), and can cause increased intestinal permeability and nutrient depletion. It can also reduce thyroid hormone usage in the body by increasing thyroid globulin. So taking the Pill can be a mixed bag. In some women it relieves cyclical mood swings, whereas in others it can amplify anxiety and depression. In some it improves acne, and in others it makes it worse. So, external regulation of hormones can have profound impacts on our body – some positive and some negative. One size does not fit all, and it is worth discussing the pros and cons of taking the contraceptive pill with your doctor.

POLYCYSTIC OVARIES

Polycystic ovaries are a common cause of fertility difficulties in women, and PCOS (polycystic ovarian syndrome) is associated with less frequent ovulation, erratic periods, weight gain and acne. It is a condition fuelled primarily by insulin resistance, so check out Chapter 8: Diabetes Discoveries if you want to understand how to minimise the effects of PCOS through diet. Generally speaking, high-fibre diets will help, as well as reducing high GI foods, such as white flour, added sugars and sugar-sweetened drinks. Anything that will improve insulin sensitivity will also be important.

Interestingly, people with PCOS tend to have more receptors for AGEs (advanced glycation end products). AGEs are proteins or fats that have a sugar attached to them – they are bio-markers associated with ageing and are present in meat, cheese, fried eggs, butter, cream and fried and heavily processed foods. When meat is cooked, especially barbecued, it releases more AGEs. So, if you minimise or cut these foods out, you can reduce the oxidative stress caused by AGEs.

Soy foods like tofu have been shown to improve PCOS – one trial from 2018 compared a standard diet of animal protein vs soy protein where the women were given the same amount of calories, protein, carbohydrate and fat. The soy group had significantly reduced body weight, waist circumference, insulin levels, insulin resistance, blood sugars and triglyceride fats in the blood.

ENDOMETRIOSIS

This is a condition where the tissue that lines the womb each month – the endometrial lining – grows and bleeds in other parts of the pelvis. With endometriosis, this endometrial lining can be found in all sorts of places – even the lungs – and the monthly bleeding can irritate and inflame, causing the potential for severe period pain, bowel loops sticking together, reduced fertility and painful sex. In severe cases, it can even result in needing to remove affected areas and a hysterectomy. It affects up to 10 per cent of women, and yet the diagnosis can be delayed by many years, either because the woman, her family or her doctor think it is just 'normal period pain'. This is primarily a diagnosis linked to excess oestrogen and, as discussed for period pain in general, a healthy plant-based diet may help. I have certainly seen it help my patients.

One study found a link between the consumption of red meat and chicken and the development of endometriosis – the women were followed up for 20 years and had had their endometriosis confirmed by laparoscopy. This suggests women who ate red meat and chicken were more at risk. This was interesting because the effect of red meat was independent of the saturated fat the women ate, and the researchers wondered if haem iron could play a part. Exposure to phthalates from plastics may be linked to endometriosis too, and interestingly foods containing the most phthalates include fish (from UK data) and chicken (from US data). More research is urgently needed as endometriosis can be a devastating diagnosis.

FIBROIDS

Inside the womb, the muscle layer can grow to form a lump, or a fibroid. Risk of fibroids increases with increasing exposure to oestrogen – interestingly, starting your periods before the age of 11 can increase the risk. This is also why fibroids tend to shrink after the menopause. If you have fibroids, you might not want to wait that long.

What do we need to know to help ourselves, as well as seeing the doctor? There is a correlation between exposure to endocrine disruptors within our fat cells and increased fibroid risk. So, losing weight helps by reducing the size of the fat cells that store these compounds, as well as by reducing the amount of oestrogen made by the fat storage cells. Perhaps unsurprisingly, fibroid lumps are associated with eating beef and ham, and one study showed green vegetables and citrus fruits are thought to be protective. Drinking

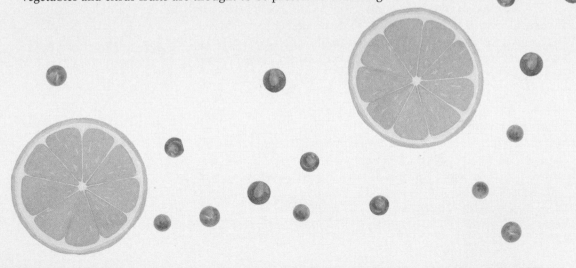

alcohol has also been linked to the development of fibroids, as well as stress and reduced physical activity. We only have observational studies at this point though, and I think more research needs to be done. However, from what has been shown so far, these lifestyle changes – eating more whole plant foods, limiting alcohol, exercising more and stressing less – are a 'nothing to lose' intervention, with everything to gain.

FERTILITY

This is a huge topic and one that cannot be covered in full. But as it is so important to many of us, I wanted to briefly mention it here.

There are many reasons why pregnancy can be hard to achieve, for some couples PCOS, fibroids or endometriosis play a part. The stress of being unable to have a baby when you desperately want one is one of life's greatest griefs. Stress can also play a big part in the struggles many couples face when they embark upon an IVF journey. I aim to emphasise to my patients how important it is to seek meaning, joy and love from other areas in your life while on the roller coaster of trying for a baby. I have seen countless couples give up on having a baby after failed fertility treatments only to fall pregnant when they least expected it, perhaps because the tension around creating life had gone, and the joy of sex had returned.

Maintaining a healthy weight is important for fertility – being overweight can stimulate oestrogen dominance and increase the risks of fibroids and PCOS. Being underweight may mean your body cannot sustain the marathon of pregnancy and childbirth. Periods can be disrupted or even stop altogether if you are not meeting your body's energy needs or if you are over-exercising. This shows you that your body is not in balance, and some changes are needed. If you are not having regular periods, discussing a return to normal monthly bleeds with your doctor will be vitally important. Weight gain or reduction, reduced exercise intensity or reduced stress will all be on the menu, and are just as important as nutrition, if not more so.

MENOPAUSE

I know, I know, menopause is a natural phase of life. Many women can sail through this transition with no symptoms. But menopause can be a very real trauma for some women, especially for those who have had to experience surgical menopause because of a hysterectomy. Hot flushes, insomnia, sexual dysfunction, vaginal dryness, mood changes and weight gain are all associated with 'the change'. Should we have to accept this as a part of life? I don't think so. There are many ways to deal with these unpleasant symptoms, and your doctor will be able to talk you through the medical treatments available, including the use of hormone replacement therapy if you choose to try it.

But could our food and lifestyle choices also make a difference?

As explained above, when women have periods, an egg is released each month, causing a surge in oestrogen and progesterone from the ovaries. But when the ovaries start running out of eggs, these hormones drop sharply too. Periods can become erratic – often by being more frequent and heavier, then becoming further apart until they stop altogether. Doctors call it menopause when you have not had a period for a year.

In case you were thinking it means the end of your 'joie de vivre' and that it's all downhill from here, I think that menopause can be a gift. Bear with me. We know that excess hormone exposure throughout our lifetime can increase our risk of developing certain cancers. What if this is nature's way of ensuring you have a better chance of a long and healthy life? Mortality rates in years gone by were skewed by childhood infections, deaths of women in childbirth and other fatal infections people sadly succumbed to – but if you made it through all that, there was actually a pretty good chance you could live to a ripe old age. Being fifty does not make you old, it marks the beginning of new possibilities, when you no longer have to look after toddlers and life can have lots more in store.

How do we make the most of menopause?

We can look to inspiration in the medical literature. A series of interviews conducted with women in the US, Canada and Japan brought interesting insights. Women in Japan tend not to have hot flushes to the same extent – or indeed even have a word for the phenomenon. The only symptoms they mentioned, other than the cessation of periods, was shoulder stiffness. Men reported this symptom about as often as the women did. Why these differences? Women were not shyer about reporting, so researchers looked towards their diets. The traditional Japanese diet is based on rice, with relatively little meat and no dairy. Japanese women were found also to be slimmer on average, meaning that the oestrogenic effect of fat cells was also minimised. Japanese women eat a lot of soy, in the form of miso soup, tofu, tempeh and edamame beans. Soy is a source of complete amino acids but also phyto-oestrogens. The isoflavones contained in soy – specifically genistein – have been shown in studies to improve menopausal symptoms, bone mineral density and reduce the risk of breast, prostate and colon cancers. One study followed Japanese women over time, and those who ate more soy were 68 per cent less likely to experience hot flushes than those who did not. Various studies have had mixed results, but it is likely that overall there may be benefit for most women.

What about popular herbal remedies? Herbal remedies can be a lifeline for many women, but results are mixed, so if you take a herbal remedy it is often a trial and error approach. Herbs with anecdotal evidence of benefits include black cohosh, red clover, ginseng, ashwaghanda, maca powder and sage leaf. However, a note of caution – the supplement industry is generally not well regulated and unless your remedy has THR (traditional herbal registration) it is hard to be sure of the concentrations and active ingredients you are getting. Always let your doctor know if you are trying something in case it interferes with another medication you are taking.

A word about HRT

A recent analysis bringing together evidence from around the world suggests that for women of average weight, five years of HRT, starting at age 50, would increase breast cancer cases by about one in 50 with combined oestrogen and progesterone, and by one in 200 with oestrogen-only HRT. These figures double after 10 years of use. Putting that into context, this translates to a roughly 2 per cent increased risk overall. This is small compared to the increased risk from obesity, regular alcohol intake and lack of exercise. For example, in post-menopausal women, the relative risk of breast cancer can increase by between 20 to 40 per cent when we carry extra weight. And three alcoholic drinks a week can increase relative risk by 15 per cent compared to women who are teetotal. So, there are risks, but putting them into the context of our lives helps, and for anyone having to deal with premature or surgical menopause, HRT can be a lifesaver. The bottom line is that every woman is different, and just as wholefoods plant-based diets are not a panacea, neither is HRT. Discuss the pros and cons with your doctor if you are not sure if it is right for you.

Men and hormones

Men go through their own hormone roller-coaster ride too. Puberty brings facial hair, voice changes, mood and muscle mass changes, and the first ejaculation. Not all bad, but certainly these changes impart a very different sense of self, and where we fit into this world. How do we make the physical side of things a little easier?

It is not just women who can be affected by weight gain and the chemicals found in plastics. Being overweight, causing higher hormone exposure, is also why men who are overweight tend to suffer from low testosterone levels and so-called 'man boobs'.

Studies have shown that reduced sperm counts, missing testes at birth (crypto-orchidism), testicular tumours and hypospadias (opening of the urethra on the underside of the penis) have all been associated with phthalate exposure. The unfortunate thing is we are exposed to these chemicals without even realising it, through all sorts of things. The list includes certain colognes and perfumes, make-up, shiny till receipts, microwave-meal wrappers and containers, plastic drinks bottles, deodorants, creams and nail polish.

Awareness is really the first step in noticing how our bodies are affected by our environment. And the great thing is, when awareness leads to action, we can gradually begin to minimise these exposures in our lives. Where we spend our money is important, because it puts pressure on manufacturers to do the right thing for us, and for the planet, by producing food, containers, make-up and body wash without these microplastics and hormone disruptors. Your wallet is just as powerful as your food choices in this sense. Buying takeaway products in compostable packaging, avoiding microwaving food in plastic or drinking from a hot plastic bottle are great ways to start limiting your plastics exposures.

SPERM COUNTS

If you have been diagnosed with a low sperm count, your doctor will advise you on the severity, and whether fertility treatments are necessary. Are there things you can do to help yourself? What can improve the quality of your little swimmers? They have a very hard job to do – each one carrying the genetic blueprint for half a human – so they have to be strong, swim in the right direction and contain healthy DNA to result in a successfully fertilised egg. What can you

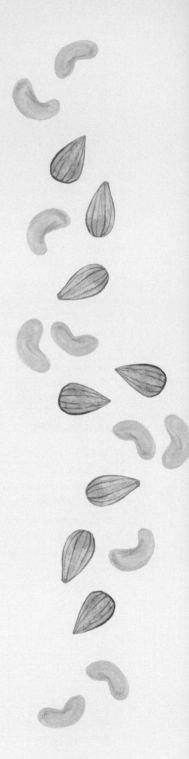

do to maximise your sperm quality? If you smoke, now is a good time to quit. If you drink heavily this is a great time to cut back too. Studies show both binge drinking and having more than fourteen drinks a week can affect sperm count and quality.

Vigorous exercise helps fertility for men and women – so long as they maintain a healthy weight. Avoiding excess heat to the testes – from cycling, tight underwear or very hot baths – may also help the sperm to survive. Limiting exposure to hormone-disrupting chemicals will be beneficial. Dioxins and heavy metals, especially concentrated in plastic-heated foods, farmed fish and processed meats, have been associated with reduced sperm quality and increased length of time to conceive. Optimising vitamin E, selenium and Co-enzyme Q10 for healthy sperm from nuts and seeds may be especially helpful. A few studies have shown an association between reduced sperm count and more saturated fat in the diet – so cutting back on meat and dairy if you are a big lover of steak and cheese may help your sperm to swim their best. Some people eat these foods twice a day or more; having them once or twice a week or less could make all the difference. Boosting low vitamin D is important – several studies link higher levels with improved sperm. Lastly, some anecdotal evidence exists for the benefits of eating fenugreek seeds to give your sperm a boost.

ERECTILE DYSFUNCTION

On the topic of sperm and fertility, I feel it is worth bringing up erections too. Although there are many causes for problems being able to sustain an erection, from psychological issues to prostate disease and low testosterone, by far the most common reason is heart disease, even in men who are in their forties. The blood vessels that lead to your penis tend to clog earlier than the ones that lead to your heart. This is an early warning sign that you are at an increased risk of heart attacks and strokes in later life. But could a plant-based diet really improve your erections? There is no doubt that fruit and vegetables and the antioxidants within them can improve blood flow, as discussed in the Chapter 5: Heart Health.

A study from Italy conducted in 2004 found that overweight men who had erectile dysfunction improved after cutting down on foods high in cholesterol (which is found only in animal products) and triglycerides (also found in oily foods). A scene from the movie *The Game Changers*, although not a scientific study, was certainly an entertaining way to show how this phenomenon might affect young men. Urologist Dr Aaron Spitz gave three elite athletes a burrito each for dinner (organic chicken, organic grass-fed beef and organic pork) and they slept with a ring device placed over the penis, in order to measure the frequency and firmness of their overnight erections. The next evening, they had a plant-based burrito dinner and repeated the test. After the plant-based meal, they had 300–500 per cent more frequent erections, which were on average four times longer in duration, harder and with a wider circumference. This certainly had the film crew and the athletes themselves convinced, but of course it does not provide definitive proof that plant-based erections are better. Perhaps you can do your own case study at home to see if this is true for you? What this data does do is point us in the direction of more plants for the win where your penis health is concerned.

SOY AND OESTROGEN

Why the fear of soy products? The name phyto-oestrogens understandably leads people to think soy products could have feminising effects, but the literature actually suggests it is a SERM (selective oestrogen receptor modulator). In other words, it acts like a weak oestrogen where it is needed and an oestrogen blocker where it is not. It turns out, this is very useful. When soy isoflavones bind to our oestrogen receptors, they provide a protective effect by improving cardiovascular health and bone strength, acting like a weak oestrogen while also reducing breast and endometrial cancer risk, acting like a weak oestrogen blocker. Put simply, it seems soy is able to provide different things depending on what your body needs. For menopausal women this is particularly useful, one study showed soy milk daily could actually increase bone mineral density compared to progesterone hormone cream and no intervention. More research is needed, but this serves as an example of how misunderstood the soy bean has been over the years . . . and as for man boobs? This is a myth. In actual fact, hops from beer are the only plant-oestrogen strong enough to have the potential for causing so called 'man boobs', also known as 'moobs'. So, to avoid man-boobs, cut out beer, not soy! My top tip is to go for minimally processed soy, such as edamame beans, tempeh, tofu and soy milk, over soy-based replacement meats.

THYROID HEALTH

The thyroid gland has an important job – it sits in the neck and regulates our body temperature and metabolism. It does its best to give you the energy you need to perform each day, and when it stops working you can develop 'hypothyroidism', or an underactive thyroid. This is usually treated with thyroid hormone supplements. If your body creates antibodies against the thyroid, you can develop a 'thyroiditis', often called Hashimotos, which results in imbalances to metabolism and body functioning. If your thyroid is overactive, you may have anxiety, sweating and a rapid pulse. Too low in function and you could feel cold, with weight gain and dry skin as symptoms.

When the thyroid is not making enough thyroid hormone, the thyroid stimulating hormone (TSH) level rises. This is because the pituitary gland in the brain is trying to stimulate the sluggish thyroid to make more hormone. What's the main reason for poor thyroid function around the world? Iodine deficiency. Iodine is crucial for thyroid function, but many soils are depleted of this mineral. This means that in some places a potato would contain plenty of iodine, but in others if the soil is not of good quality, there are negligible amounts. In the US, salt is iodised, making deficiency relatively rare. That is not the case in the UK. Iodine is found in cow's milk because it is used in sanitising agents for milk storage units and is also given in the feed of cows who provide milk. If you don't drink cow's milk, fortunately there are now many iodine supplemented multivitamins and fortified plant milks available – but you will have to check the label.

Seaweed is a natural source of iodine. In fact, I like to think of seaweed as 'sea plants'. Sea plants are a sustainable and healthy way to get nutrients we may miss out on now we are living with the consequences of overfishing and industrial toxin exposures in our oceans. They are not subject to the same concentration of toxins because they are further down the food chain. A typical sheet of dried nori, used for making sushi but really tasty as a snack by itself, is a source of iodine, containing about 40mcg of it in a large sheet. Iodine is a goldilocks mineral though – too little is harmful, but so is too much. Eating large amounts of seaweeds like kelp – which can be very high in iodine – is a bad idea for this reason. If you want to keep things simple, I would generally recommend choosing a non-seaweed iodine supplement containing no more than 150mcg of iodine in the form of 'potassium iodide' or 'potassium iodate'.

Selenium is another important mineral to keep the hormonal melodies in tune – we need iodine and selenium working together to keep the thyroid happy. It helps protect the thyroid from oxidative stress by making an antioxidant called glutathione. And selenium helps in activating thyroid hormone (converting T4 to T3 in the body). Plant-based sources of selenium are Brazil nuts, brown rice, wholegrain spaghetti and pasta, beans and seeds – luckily you only need one Brazil nut a day and you should be covered. Maximise phenylalanine in your food to help thyroid hormone production – this is found in beans, nuts, seeds, wholemeal pasta, wholegrain bread and veggies like sweet potatoes.

Zinc helps to stimulate the production of thyroid hormone too – if you are minimising animal products it can be found in seeds, nuts, beans, tofu, wholegrains, lentils and brown rice. To boost uptake further, these foods can be fermented, soaked or sprouted. And garlic can be added to help boost your absorption of zinc. Why not blend it in your hummus or rice?

Finally, iron is needed to allow TPO (thyroid peroxidase) to stimulate the production of thyroid hormones. Plant-based sources of iron include wholegrains, lentils, chickpeas, beans, pumpkin seeds and dried fruit. Tomato sauces can take up iron from cast-iron cookware too.

THYROID HEALTH ON A WFPB DIET

There is not much data on the benefits of a WFPB diet for thyroid function. Some epidemiological data suggests that plant-based diets are associated with lower rates of hypothyroidism. Other research shows us how beneficial plant-based diets can be for reducing the risk of various autoimmune diseases. What is clear is that iodine levels must be adequate – or else the whole hormonal harmony will be off balance. This will make the body more susceptible to the effects of iodine-uptake blocking foods like soy and cruciferous vegetables. Cooking can deactivate the enzymes involved, but crucially, ensuring you have enough iodine and selenium in your diet will be the most important thing you can do to ensure you can use all these healthy plant compounds in the right way.

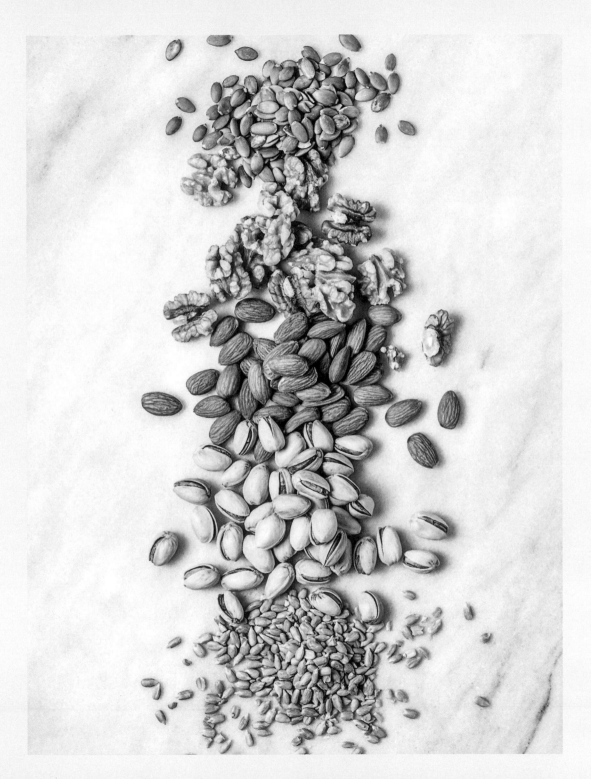

- Cut back on processed foods because they tend to have higher levels of unhealthy fats and other exposures not great for hormonal health.

- Eat more plant-based foods so you have plenty of fibre to boost hormonal regulation.

- Try fermented foods to feed your gut buddies, such as tempeh, miso and sauerkraut.

- Enjoy minimally processed soy every day, especially if you are menopausal. But if you have a thyroid imbalance, speak to your doctor or dietician, as you may need to modify the amount or eat it at different times from your thyroid hormone supplement.

- Eat a handful of nuts every day (walnuts, peeled almonds, or macadamias) or some avocado for healthy fats. These are vital for the absorption of fat-soluble vitamins like vitamins A, D, E and K.

- Sprinkle two tablespoons of ground flax seeds on your food daily for healthy omega-3 fats.

- Use herbs and spices like turmeric, ginger, sage, parsley, mint and cardamom in your food – they are packed full of antioxidants and polyphenols. Fenugreek may help with the flow of breast milk and sperm quality in men too.

- Herbal teas are your friend – a lovely way of getting more antioxidants while also curbing appetite when you get the evening munchies.

- Eat tryptophan-rich foods like oats, pumpkin seeds, squash and soy.

- Limit sugar-sweetened drinks, refined flour and bread.

- Prioritise fruit as a snack and a healthy natural sugar.

- Curb the booze.

- Minimise plastics exposures in your food and drink by avoiding heating food in plastic and using plastic-free containers.

- Move your body – this gets the lymph flowing and improves fertility if not exercising to excess.

- Make sure that you consume enough magnesium because it plays an essential role in hormone regulation. It regulates cortisol, so calms the nervous system by balancing hormone levels, including progesterone, oestrogen and testosterone. Foods that are rich in magnesium include green leafy vegetables, almonds, legumes and dark chocolate.

- Eat a multitude of fruits and veggies to give you plenty of vitamin C, beta-carotene for vitamin A, vitamins B2, B3 and B6. Aim to include smoothies, salads, fruit snacks and steamed vegetables in your daily diet.

- Check your vitamin D is in the normal range, and if not, grab a vitamin D3 supplement. Most, if not all of us, can benefit from a supplement in winter months. I talk more about this in Part Two.

- B12 supplements are a must if you are fully plant-based, and vitamin D3 and EPA/DHA supplements from algae oil supplements may also be helpful to add to your routine.

CASE STUDY – SHELLY'S STORY

There are some days when I get an unexpected surprise: a person who decides they are so ready for change that they will seek it through the smallest of nudges. That's what happened to Shelly. She was a 48-year-old woman who had come in tearful and desperate. Shelly was getting severe period cramps as well as hot flushes and frequent episodes of anxiety. She was tired all the time and would regularly wake in the early hours of the morning in a panic. She described it as two weeks of hell every month in which the cramps were unbearable with breast tenderness too. She was not a medication person; she admitted that she was not likely to take any treatments, and we had already done the standard blood tests to rule out things like thyroid imbalances. She was 'peri-menopausal', so in the limbo land of still having periods but also experiencing crippling symptoms of menopause. She was not depressed or lacking in purpose, and there were no major stressors at the root of her problems. I decided to talk about simple lifestyle measures that could improve her symptoms. I briefly explained that a WFPB eating pattern may help. She was sceptical. She told me she already had a healthy lifestyle.

'I really don't see how this could help me, doctor,' she said.

Shelly really felt she had tried everything. I understood – she was avoiding junk food and getting regular exercise, so perhaps there was nothing more she could do. However, unbeknown to me, she bought a plant-based cookbook. She cooked the recipes. She began to conduct her own online research. She decided to eat tofu or edamame beans every day as I had suggested this may help her flushes. Her mood swings began to subside. Her periods became lighter and she experienced no cramping at all. The breast tenderness had gone and she began to sleep very well. Her anxiety had also gone. She came into my consultation room beaming, saying, 'I feel as though I look younger, the bagginess around my eyes has disappeared too!'

Ten months later, she had lost around 9lb in weight without trying, and no longer got any bloating. Crucially, she had so much more energy. She was confident, happy and truly vibrant.

Everyone is unique, and it's rarely one thing that 'fixes' us. But Shelly's sense of gratitude, her transformation and her newfound vibrancy were too special not to share. And it taught me – and her – a valuable lesson. Never lose hope that you can feel better than you currently do. Even at the worst of times, there is a new perspective to be found. In this case, plant-based eating was just the change in perspective that she needed.

A HEALTHY GUT

It is more than just you living in your body – we have trillions of micro-organisms – bacteria, viruses, fungi and other life forms residing in each of us, and these organisms are collectively known as the microbiome. These outnumber our human cells by ten to one. In fact, we have more bugs living within us than there are stars in our galaxy. Just think about how awe-inspiring that is.

So, it stands to reason that we are not just eating for our health, but for them too! Various organs have different microbial residents and the area which has attracted the most attention over the last 15 years is the gut microbiome. We now understand that everything that goes on our plates, from a serving of broccoli to a slice of beef, has an effect on this incredible population of micro-organisms.

Gut health is widely considered the next frontier of health and well-being, and evidence continues to mount around the importance of our gut bugs and the link between them and our health. We know that the gut microbiome affects the body from before birth and determines not only the digestion of the food that we consume but a host of systems, including our immune system, our central nervous system and our risk of obesity, cancer and chronic disease.

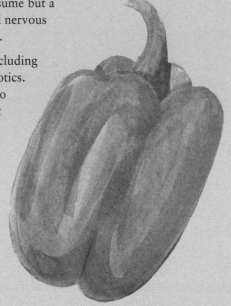

There are many factors that affect our gut microbiome, including (but not limited to) our environments, genetics and antibiotics. Many of these things cannot be changed. However, we also know diet plays a significant role and even though our gut microbiota is relatively stable, what we eat in just 24 hours can change our microbiome, for better or worse. Our food choices can significantly impact our gut microbiota and modern lifestyles, including a Western diet, have led to substantial depletion of gut microbial diversity.

What keeps our microbiome diverse? Eating as many different types of fruits, vegetables, wholegrains and legumes as we can. Some worry that a WFPB approach will restrict them, when in fact it introduces a much broader range of different foods for our microbiome than the same staples from a standard Western diet.

Links have been made with obesity and critical diseases like colorectal cancer. A lack of diversity of gut bugs has also been shown in people with chronic conditions, including diabetes, irritable bowel syndrome (IBS), coeliac disease, Alzheimer's and psoriatic arthritis.

A diverse microbiome is important because it helps to deter bacteria that can make us unwell, and it can keep our population of gut bugs more stable and resilient if we are ill. One study from 2019 found that following a healthy WFPB diet for about four months can boost your gut microbiome diversity and lead to improvements in body weight and blood sugar management. Researchers studied 147 participants, randomised into two groups. One followed a low-fat vegan diet. The other group made no changes to their diet. After the 16-week study was completed, researchers reported that the vegan group saw their body weight, fat mass and visceral fat levels fall. Changes to their gut microbiome were swift too, which is what surprised the researchers the most.

Is there any evidence on how animal foods can affect our gut? Saturated fats, which are found predominantly in animal products, can weaken the gut lining. They cause an imbalance of gut bacteria, which opens the tight junctions that create the normal barrier protecting our gut from pathogens. The dying bacteria release LPS (lipopolysaccharides) from their cell walls. These are endotoxins which cause inflammation within our bodies. Another link found by a cardiologist is the metabolite TMAO. Trimethylamine N-oxide (TMAO) increases risk of heart disease, heart failure and chronic kidney disease. It is formed in your body as bacteria in your gut help digest the choline and carnitine provided by meat, eggs, fish and chicken. Interestingly, research is showing this only happens when we have cultivated the bugs needed to digest meat – if you feed a vegan a beef steak their TMAO blood levels remain low. So, although this is only one factor in health, the research shows us that restoring our gut's balance and ensuring diversity is a crucial factor in preventing and treating chronic diseases.

HOW TO KEEP OUR GUT BUGS HAPPY

Once we have a happy house of beneficial microbes, what can we do to keep them happy? In one word: **fibre**.

Food travels to our small intestine where it is metabolised, digested and absorbed, ready to be used as energy. When we eat fibre, it makes its way through the small intestine and into the large intestine, undigested and intact. The large intestine is home to most of the gut microbes that break down this fibre.

Certain 'protective' bacteria digest fibre, producing short-chain fatty acids (SCFAs), which are the by-products of the fermentation of food by gut bugs. But they are very important by-products. SCFAs protect against inflammation (see pages 130–31) and play a key role in immunity.

Fibre plays a vital role in keeping the gut and digestive system healthy by helping the muscles in your small and large intestines to work properly and move your stools through your body. It 'sweeps' along and clears harmful compounds, unwanted hormones and toxins so they cannot be reabsorbed into our bloodstreams and into our tissues. Fibre also adds bulk and softens stools to relieve constipation and can prevent and relieve problems such as haemorrhoids or piles, diverticulitis and irritable bowel syndrome (IBS). There is also evidence that eating a diet high in fibre reduces the risk of developing serious conditions such as diabetes, heart disease and some kinds of cancers, especially bowel cancer. One meta-analysis suggests that every 10g of fibre we eat per day cuts our premature mortality risk by an amazing 10 per cent.

One of the main ways in which fibre can reduce cancer and early death rates is its important role in helping us to maintain a healthy weight. As mentioned before, fibre will keep you fuller for longer, but without adding empty calories. It can also help those who are overweight to lose excess pounds. This weight loss reduces our risk of developing chronic disease.

Fibre falls into two main categories and both are beneficial to our health:

Soluble fibre dissolves in water and is broken down by natural bacteria in your bowels. It can lower glucose and cholesterol levels in the blood. Foods that contain soluble fibre include oats, barley and pulses.

Insoluble fibre does not dissolve but attracts water and travels through your body mostly unchanged. It acts like a broom and helps to move food through your digestive system, promoting bowel health. It also supports insulin sensitivity, so may reduce the risk of diabetes. Foods which contain insoluble fibre include fruit and vegetables with skin and pips, as well as nuts and wholegrain cereals like wheat, rice and rye.

Most fruit and vegetables contain a combination of soluble and insoluble fibre. Animal products do not contain any fibre and refined grains like white bread contain less fibre than unrefined wholegrains. So, the more you replace meat and refined grains like white flour with WFPB meals, the more space you have for fibre in your diet. When you start to increase the amount of fibre you eat, it is important to drink plenty of water too, because these fibres dissolve in, and draw water to them. It can therefore cause constipation if there is not enough water to go around.

In the UK, only 1 in 10 adults make the recommended fibre intake of 30g per day. When we eat fibre, our gut bugs make compounds that crush inflammation and help defend us against infection as well as keeping us full. Even though this is the recommended amount, I would suggest that the more fibre we eat, the better. A WFPB diet will be naturally high in fibre, so you won't need to think about how many grams you are getting every day.

How can we help our guts? The best way to start is to ditch processed foods, animal protein and saturated fat, and instead focus on a plant-based, minimally processed high-fibre diet.

Foods that make our gut particularly happy include:

- Ginger
- Garlic
- Bananas
- Brussel sprouts
- Peas
- Almonds

- Kimchi
- Sauerkraut
- Artichokes
- Cauliflower
- Broccoli
- Okra

- Yams
- Gherkins
- Leeks
- Asparagus

A NOTE ABOUT PROBIOTICS AND PREBIOTICS

Many patients ask me about probiotics and their potential benefits, and the answer is not straightforward. This is an unregulated industry. One popular use is to replenish the gut after a course of antibiotics. The logic is that antibiotics wipe out your beneficial gut bacteria along with the harmful bacteria, so by taking probiotics, you can replenish your microbiome.

Saccharomyces boulardii is a bacteria often given for preventing and treating diarrhoea in the form of probiotic tablets. The evidence is mixed, and we still do not know the long-term effects of taking probiotics. Some research has even shown that they can delay gut-health recovery.

There are some studies that show they are helpful in some cases, but their benefits are short-lived. I like to think of it as the cavalry coming charging through – but they do not stick around and are ultimately pooped out. Long-term microbiome health comes from fibre and a WFPB diet. Remember diversity is key, rather than creating limited amounts of one or two types of bug through tablets, however beneficial they seem. I encourage you to get your good bugs from diet and not pills.

Have you heard of prebiotics? Prebiotics are defined as 'non-digestible food that benefits the host by selectively stimulating the growth and activity of bacteria in the colon.' They have been touted as helping a huge range of conditions from obesity to mental health. But what are prebiotics really? Fibre! Food for our gut bugs and for us. Getting us back to our fruits and veggies means we feed the gut bugs we already have, tending to that intestinal garden in the best possible way.

A NOTE ABOUT ANTIBIOTICS

When they were first introduced in 1944, antibiotics were considered a miracle cure. And they are, after all, because before they came along even the smallest of scratches could prove fatal. But in order to ensure they still work, they need to be used sparingly.

Antimicrobial resistance (AMR), particularly antibiotic resistance, is one of the greatest threats to our health. This is where infections become resistant to antibiotics. In the UK, AMR has been put on the government's national risk register alongside terrorism and pandemic flu.

Public Health England recently announced there are 165 new antibiotic-resistant infections every day in the UK. It's scary stuff. As doctors, we used to imagine that all infections could be dealt with, as long as we knew what bug was growing. Now, there is a very real fear that routine surgeries could become a thing of the past and procedures such as Caesareans could present so many more risks as a result of our misuse of antibiotics.

In my clinic, like all doctors, we aim to educate and inform about when antibiotics may not be needed and in some cases may harm.

But don't forget that antibiotics can still affect you even if you have not taken a course of antibiotics yourself. Antibiotics are given extensively to animals bred for farming around the globe. In some countries such as the US (though not the UK), they are used in low doses to prevent disease and promote growth. In the UK, they are used to treat infections. According to the Soil Association, intensively reared pigs and poultry account for 79 per cent of UK farming antibiotic use. If you eat pork and chicken often, you could be consuming antibiotic-resistant bacteria with every meal.

The UN predicts that antibiotic resistance will account for 10 million extra deaths by 2050. When most of this is being driven by the meat and dairy industry, we have to seriously think about what we choose to eat and drink.

If you eat meat, I advise you to think of it as more of a 'sometimes food' and keep portions small (see page 59). Aim to buy free-range and organic, where the routine use of antibiotics is banned. This is more expensive but plant protein sources such as lentils, beans and chickpeas are much cheaper.

DIVERTICULITIS

The healthy colon has an inner and an outer layer. Normally, these layers squeeze and relax together to allow digested food to flow through the gut, and then it gets pushed out through our bottoms as poo. Pressure can build up when the poo gets hard and gets stuck. That pressure gets worse when we strain to get the poo out. When this happens, the inner layer of the intestine pushes through weak spots in the outer layer, and makes balloons of intestine herniate, or push out. These balloons, or pouches, are known as diverticula. They are most commonly found in the lower part of the large intestine on the left-hand side, but they can appear anywhere in the gut. Between 30 to 50 per cent of people in the Western world will develop diverticular disease and it is more common as we get older. 'Diverticulosis' is the name for having all these stretched pockets of gut, and 'diverticulitis' is what we call it when the pockets with stagnant poo get inflamed and infected. Sometimes there will be no symptoms, but occasionally it can cause severe abdominal pain, fever, nausea and even bowel obstruction and perforation.

Most people suffering from diverticulitis are normally recommended a low-fibre diet but there is little evidence for its effectiveness. If a diverticulitis flare-up is mild, I advise my patients to let the gut rest and drink fluids and eat foods like soup for a while. This is because a low-roughage diet will avoid spasm of the gut as it is trying to work against the blockage and infection. Some people may also need antibiotics. But once symptoms have eased, high-fibre foods are crucial to get the gut moving normally again. The more fibre we eat, the softer and bulkier our stools will be. Many studies have shown that eating fibre-rich foods can control diverticular symptoms.

INFLAMMATORY BOWEL DISEASE (IBD)

IBD should not be confused with irritable bowel syndrome (IBS), which is a different diagnosis. IBD causes severe gut inflammation and ulceration and there are two main types: Crohn's disease and ulcerative colitis. Symptoms can be horrible: diarrhoea, weight loss, stomach cramps and blood or mucous in the stools. In Crohn's disease, healthy parts of the intestine are mixed with inflamed areas and it can affect any part of the digestive tract. In ulcerative colitis, inflammation and ulceration occurs in the lining of the colon and rectum. People who have IBD have a depleted mucous layer in their bowel, and bacteria passes through the cell junctions, causing the immune system to go into overdrive.

Living with Crohn's or ulcerative colitis is hard, and flare-ups can disrupt everyday life, sometimes even requiring life-changing surgery. There is no cure. Only about 10 per cent of patients with Crohn's disease achieve long-term remission, and many people live with ongoing symptoms. Half of all patients require surgery within ten years of being diagnosed. This is shocking. My patients with IBD should not have to live this way.

Why is IBD becoming so much more common, and what can we do about it? We know that high-fat, low-fibre and animal-heavy diets can worsen these problems. More research is being done in this area but we know that cutting out processed foods, emulsifiers and meat, and increased intake of dietary fibre is beneficial. Study after study in animal models have shown that a diet high in saturated fat causes an unhealthy balance in the microbiota, impairs intestinal barrier function, and leads to the release of bacterial endotoxin. A recent case study has also shown a man with Crohn's disease achieved complete remission within six months of following a WFPB diet. A fibre-filled approach also seems to reduce the risk of developing Crohn's in the first place. The Harvard Nurse's Study, involving over 120,000 women, showed that women with a higher fibre intake had a 40 per cent reduced risk of developing Crohn's.

Why? Soluble fibre reduces inflammation in the bowel and helps to maintain the integrity of the gut lining, or epithelial barrier. It is also thought that the phytonutrients in fibre-rich foods help to protect the bowel. Lastly, and perhaps most importantly, we come back to the effect of fibre on our gut microbiota. You see, the destruction of our gut bugs also plays a part in how and whether fibre can help us at all.

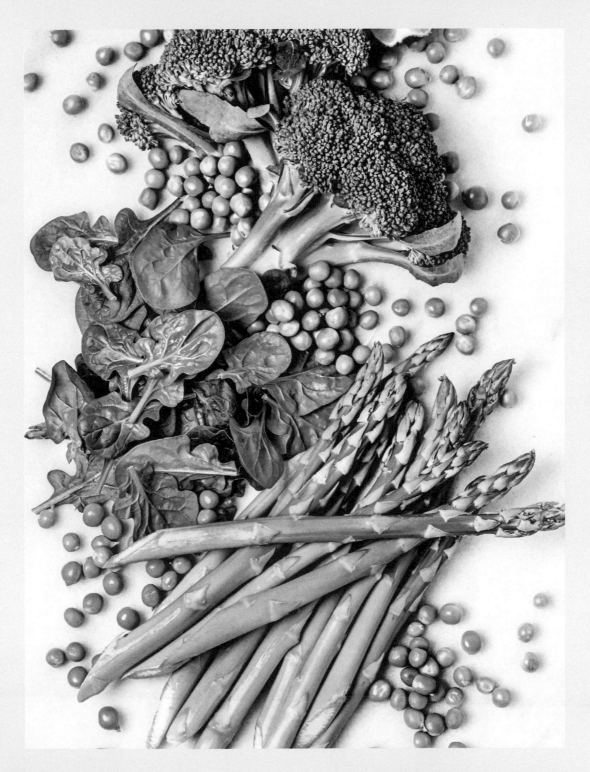

Bloating and discomfort is common when we are not used to increasing our fibre intake, and this can be eased when we introduce these foods more gradually, giving our guts a chance to heal. It allows time to bring in the right bugs to help digest fibre properly. With a damaged gut lining, and without the right gut bugs in the right place in the gut, immune system mediated conditions such as inflammatory bowel disease, coeliac disease, asthma, eczema and inflammatory arthritis are all on the rise.

Our modern world is not helping us out here. Pesticides, antibiotics, alcohol, poor sleep, air pollution and fast food can all play a detrimental role. It is clear when we look at the relationship between our inner ecosystem of trillions of gut bugs and our external ecosystem, that our internal and external environments are all far more connected than we could ever have imagined.

One great step towards healing the gut and the immune system is to choose fibre-rich plant foods. A bonus is if you can get them grown with minimal pesticides and close to where you live. Thankfully, following a WFPB approach will means you will be getting plenty of fibre.

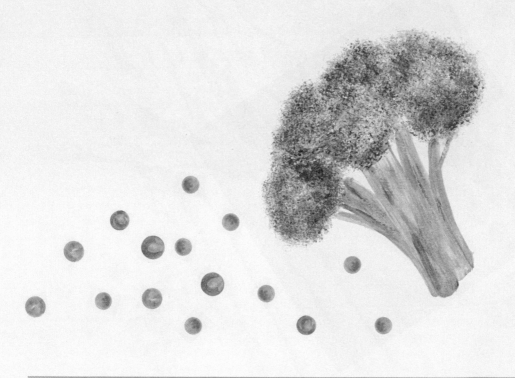

TOP TIPS FOR IMPROVING GUT HEALTH

Avoid mouthwash

Avoiding the use of mouthwash, but instead flossing and brushing your tongue and teeth properly, will do wonders for your mouth microbiome. Remember, your gastro-intestinal tract runs from your mouth to your bottom, so stripping your mouth of the beneficial microbes you need to help you digest your vegetables can actually reduce the amount of nitric oxide your blood vessels can make. This fascinating link may explain why in a handful of studies mouthwash use has been linked to increased risk of diabetes and high blood pressure.

Limit alcohol

Just as alcohol was used to sterilise surgical equipment back in the day, so too will your gut bugs be stripped when you overdo the booze. Alcohol reduces your ability to gain nutrition from food, particularly thiamine, B12, folic acid and zinc.

Don't eat late

Late-night eating disrupts the circadian rhythm of your gut bugs as well as spiking your blood sugar. Your gut microbiome and digestive enzymes tend to work best if you eat your largest meal in the middle of the day.

Relax

Stress can have an effect on your gut microbiome. New research shows that social stress, such as loneliness, alters both the composition and behaviour of gut bacteria.

Sleep well

If you suffer from insomnia, your microbiome shifts towards bacterial populations that promote obesity.

Move your body

Moving outside is even better! Studies show being in urban environments is detrimental to gut bugs and being in nature helps rebalance your biome so why not combine movement with being outside? Believe it or not, exercise can diversify your gut flora and increase your butyrate levels (one of the short-chain fatty acids that your gut bugs love).

Clean with care
Bleach, harsh cleaning products and antibacterial washes can leave skin feeling dry and strip you of beneficial microbes on the outside of your body. Washing your hands with soap and drying them is just as effective – without the exposure to chemicals that disrupt your skin biome.

Cautious use of medications
Take care when taking medications: antibiotics, NSAIDs (anti-inflammatories such as ibuprofen and naproxen), and oral contraceptives can be particularly problematic for our gut microbes and the integrity of our gut lining.

Avoid white bread and sugar
Highly processed white bread, pasta and sugary cereals reduce our beneficial gut-bug diversity and cause a rise in inflammatory bacteria which can then drive sugar cravings.

Steer clear of emulsifiers
Aim to avoid emulsifiers such as carboxymethylcelluose, polysorbate 80 and carrageenan. Never heard of them? They are in a fair amount of processed foods and plant milks, so always check the label.

Ditch the sweeteners
Although more research is needed, artificial sweeteners like aspartame, sucralose, xylitol and trehalose could all adversely affect our gut microbiome and trehalose may increase populations of harmful bug C. difficile, which is a cause of severe colitis.

Eat prebiotics
Foods such as garlic, leeks, oats, bananas, lentils, chickpeas and beans are packed with prebiotics. Your gut bugs love them!

Ferment for the win
Sauerkraut, miso, kimchi and tempeh are all examples of fermented foods that will benefit your gut.

CASE STUDY – JACQUI'S STORY

Jacqui is a patient of mine who had developed Crohn's disease, as well as a liver disease called primary sclerosing cholangitis, kidney disease, and asthma. You'll notice that all her conditions were affecting different organs – the lungs, the liver and gallbladder, the kidneys and the gut. But there was a commonality with these conditions too; they were affected by her immune responses, and in some cases caused by them.

When she first came in to see me, she was desperate. It was her Crohn's disease that was bothering her most. She was getting a lot of abdominal pain and was finding that as a result of her unpredictable bowel motions, she could barely leave the house. Any time she made plans with her friends, she had to cancel them because her gut was so unpredictable. She was in her early 60s but felt as though her life was over. We talked a lot about the things she wanted to do. Jacqui felt her life was governed by hospital appointments and yet, despite all her medications and the hospital specialists who were taking such good care of her, she sat in front of me on the verge of tears.

What could I offer her? I felt stumped. But something she had not tried, despite eating healthily all her life, was a WFPB diet. She gave it a go.

'I've got nothing to lose,' she'd said to me. What I realised then, and to this day, is that any change in lifestyle has to come from the individual making the choice to change, not from the person suggesting it. I was in the right place at the right time.

When she came back to see me for a kidney disease follow-up appointment, she looked energised and radiant. I knew something had shifted in her before she had even sat down. She couldn't wait to share the good news with me. When she made the switch, she said one of the first things she noticed was that she was not bloated any more. She also noticed she had a lot less tummy pain, and crucially for her social plans, she did not need to run to the toilet all the time!

'I feel so much better in myself!' she exclaimed.

When I asked her if she needed any more inhalers from her prescription, she said, 'Well, you can give them to me if you want, but I don't seem to need them like I used to, doctor.'

'OK . . .' I replied. 'Well, what about your kidney function, shall we check that?'

'You can do,' she replied, 'But the kidney specialist has actually discharged me now, so I must be doing all right . . .'

When I reviewed her hospital correspondence, her kidney specialist seemed shocked that her kidney function readings were so good. He brought her back to clinic twice, and as she had maintained normal kidney function over those months, he had discharged her from follow up. And, the best news of all, her Crohn's disease had improved so much that she had also been discharged from follow up by her Crohn's specialist too.

Jacqui had gone from a woman whose existence was filled with hospital appointments, medications and symptoms that disrupted her life, to a woman who could live her life more fully than ever before. She was absolutely delighted and, of course, so was I.

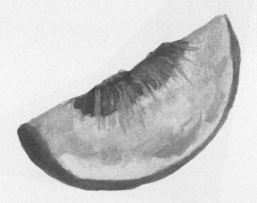

THE PLANT POWER DOCTOR

IMMUNITY

A healthy immune system fights germs, cancers and other threats to the body. Autoimmune conditions develop when our immune system mistakenly attacks healthy tissue, leading to inflammation (see pages 26–8). There are more than 80 different types of autoimmune conditions; I have already covered some, such as Type 1 diabetes and inflammatory bowel disease, but other common autoimmune illnesses include lupus, rheumatoid arthritis, MS and psoriasis. These diseases are often hard to diagnose and can manifest themselves in a variety of symptoms, and they are also on the rise.

While genetic and environmental factors play a role, and infections – especially viral – are thought to be a major trigger of autoimmune disease, the truth is that we still have much to understand about why these processes happen, and what is at the root of them. Autoimmune disease labels can be really frustrating from a patient's point of view, and from my experience can be tremendously disempowering. We are telling our patients their bodies cannot be trusted, we do not know why this has happened and, when they are sent from specialist to specialist without a resolution of their symptoms, they are often left feeling broken and that there's nothing they can do to get better.

However, there is a growing body of evidence that lifestyle factors, including a WFPB diet, can positively impact, or sometimes even completely reverse, some autoimmune conditions. These diseases can be frustrating and hard to manage during flare-ups, but food can be a powerful tool in helping your body fight back. Do not be afraid to dream, and to imagine a healthier and happier version of yourself. If you are afraid to hope, you are afraid to act.

So, let's go over some of the reasons why a wholefoods plant-based approach could be helpful when we have an autoimmune condition.

Reduces inflammation

Dietary triggers may play an inciting role in the autoimmune process, and a compromised intestinal barrier may allow food components or micro-organisms to enter the bloodstream, triggering inflammation. Diets high in fat and processed meat are associated with higher inflammatory markers, such as C-reactive protein (CRP) whereas WFPB diets have been associated with lower levels. Reducing inflammation is critical to good health.

Lowers BMI

WFPB diets are also associated with a lower BMI, and lower body weight reduces the risk of developing rheumatoid arthritis. One 2018 analysis found that RA patients who lost more than 5kg of body weight were three times more likely to experience improvements than those who lost less than 5kg.

Heals the gut

I have discussed how the gut plays an important role in immunity. Gut health is a crucial component when it comes to healing and preventing the development of autoimmune disease. WFPB diets promote healthy gut bacteria and diversity of the microbiome, which is often lacking in patients with arthritis.

Remember why gut health is so foundational to immune health? Just beyond the wall of your intestine sits 70 per cent of your immune system. When infections or even cancerous cells come to the attention of immune cells, it is their job to figure out which ones to kill and which to leave alone.

How do you separate friend from foe when there are millions of microbes in the gut mingling with your food and drink, which contain pesticides, metals, plastics, bacteria, viruses and fungi of their own, not to mention the 30 trillion human cells they will meet too? That's a lot to deal with. Too vigorous a response and you get allergic or autoimmune issues. Too laid-back and you get infections or even cancer.

How do we help the immune system figure things out? What can translate the message into a language the immune cells understand? The short-chain fatty acids (SCFAs) produced from fibre do a great job as translator (see page 117).

Fruit, vegetables, wholegrains and legumes get broken down into these SCFAs by gut microbes, and the immune response to SCFAs is to relax. In fact, SCFAs have been shown to inhibit three of the most powerful inflammatory signallers in the body. This is important not just for dealing with immune disorders, but also for potentially reducing food sensitivities over time.

RHEUMATOID ARTHRITIS

There is evidence that a WFPB diet can alleviate the symptoms of rheumatoid arthritis. A clinical trial on 24 people that looked at the effects of a low-fat vegan diet on people with moderate-to-severe rheumatoid arthritis found that after just four weeks on the diet, participants experienced significant improvements in morning stiffness, pain, joint tenderness and joint swelling. Although this is a small study, it guides future research. It has also been noted that a WFPB diet is packed with nutrients that can support and help to balance immunity, including potassium, fibre, vitamins A, C and K, magnesium and beta-carotene.

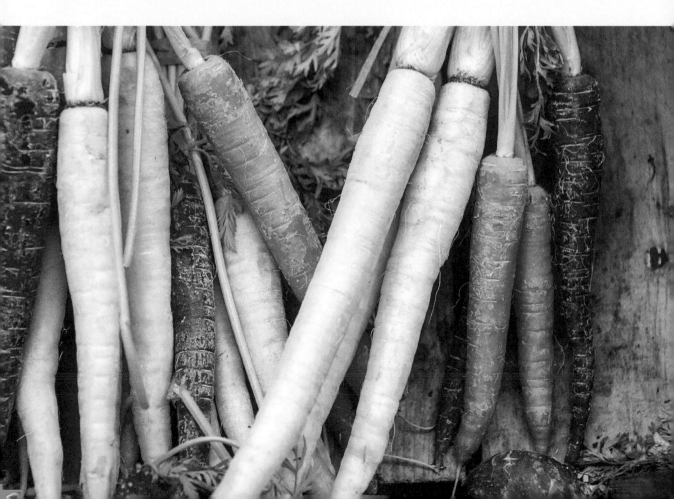

CASE STUDY – IIDA'S STORY

Iida, who was in her early 30s, had been suffering from knee pain that left her in agony and unable to walk on occasion. Standing up for more than a few minutes resulted in severe swelling and pain. She visited osteopaths and physiotherapists and, after seven months of investigations under a rheumatologist, she was diagnosed with inflammatory arthritis. She experienced severe side effects from the medication she was prescribed, which saw her ending up in A&E. Her rheumatologist told her she was likely to be on medication for the rest of her life to try to control the symptoms of her condition. She turned to the internet, desperate to find a way to improve her symptoms. After discovering a rheumatoid arthritis support group online, she overhauled her diet. She started by cutting out dairy, sugar and gluten, and immediately noticed a difference.

A month later, she stopped eating meat and oils. Her body responded quickly and within two weeks her test results came back as normal. She combined her WFPB diet with other lifestyle exercises, such as yoga, and she is now completely symptom free. She has found the most exciting aspect of her healing has been her ability to have drug and pain-free pregnancies, in stark contrast to early predictions based on her autoimmune condition. She now has a son and daughter and years later remains well and without joint inflammation.

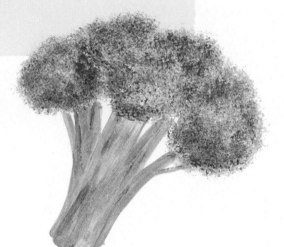

LUPUS

Lupus (or SLE, systemic lupus erythematosus) is a long-term autoimmune condition, where the body's immune system goes into overdrive and attacks normal and healthy tissue. Symptoms can include inflammation, swelling, and damage to joints, blood, kidneys, heart and lungs. It is complex and presents itself in many ways, so can be hard to diagnose. As with arthritis, a WFPB diet can help to alleviate symptoms.

CASE STUDY – DR BROOKE GOLDNER'S STORY

Dr Brooke Goldner is one of the best-known doctors in the practical application of dietary change to treat lupus. Diagnosed with lupus at the age of 16, she went on to suffer from advanced kidney failure and was told she may only have six months to live. She spent two years on chemotherapy to control her condition. For the next decade, she struggled to control her symptoms and experienced blood clots and mini strokes. After adopting a WFPB diet, her lupus was gone within four months. She was able to have two successful pregnancies despite her prognosis and is now in her forties and healthier than ever.

Dr Goldner has dedicated her career to helping others do the same through her basic emphasis on hydration, 'hyper-nourishment' with foods such as cruciferous veggies, green smoothies and plant-based omega-3s. Although much more research is needed on this topic, animal studies have shown benefits with vitamins A, D, E, phyto-oestrogens and polyunsaturated fatty acids (PUFAs), and patient studies have also shown benefits from reducing calories in general, so as to avoid being overweight. There is no doubt that nutrition has a role to play in the management of lupus, and in the prevention of its complications.

MULTIPLE SCLEROSIS

MS is an unpredictable degenerative condition in which the immune system destroys myelin – the fatty substance that surrounds nerve fibres in the brain and spine. It often strikes in the prime of life and symptoms include fatigue, and problems with vision, tremors, pain and paralysis. For many, this diagnosis can feel devastating, but there is hope.

A distinguished neurologist called Dr Roy Swank looked at MS data during the Second World War and noted the reduced rate of MS when meat and dairy were rationed. One of his studies found that MS strongly correlated with the amount of saturated animal fat eaten. He decided to put it to the test and asked his own MS patients to cut their saturated animal fat so that it made up about 10 per cent of what they ate – incredibly he was able to publish their results after 3, 5, 7, 20 and even 34 years follow up. This is extremely rare. Altogether, 144 patients made it to the 34 years follow up. What he found was that in those who had early disease, this strategy seemed to stop progression in its tracks, with 95 per cent of them having no further disability 34 years later. In those who increased their saturated fat intake, even after many years without symptoms, their disability and mortality risks went back up. So dietary change helped, but only for as long as they kept the same habits day to day. To date, no medication or intervention has come close to achieving these results. One pilot study examined the effects of a low-fat, vegan diet with MS progression, disease activity and quality of life. Sixty-one participants with MS were followed for a year. About half adhered to a very low-saturated fat, WFPB eating plan. While the study resulted in no significant improvement on brain MRIs, there were significant improvements in relapse rates, with lower disability and fatigue scores in those who ate plant-based foods. They had better ability to function day to day and more energy. Participants were also able to lose weight and reduce cholesterol levels and they also had higher scores in quality of life and overall mood. Larger studies are needed, but these results are hugely promising.

CASE STUDY – DR SARAY STANCIC AND DR CONOR KERLEY'S STORY

Dr Saray Stancic and Dr Conor Kerley are just two of many doctors and dieticians who decided to apply the research to their own lives when they developed MS.

Dr Stancic was a young, energetic physician when she developed sudden paralysis as she was getting up for a call from the ER. After eight years of symptoms she stumbled upon a piece of research that was set to change her life, a research article on the benefits of blueberries. This began a deep dive into nutritional science and how it related to MS.

She began her journey into WFPB eating back in 2003, and now her focus is on educating her patients about lifestyle medicine as a result of her research and experiences of disease remission.

Dr Kerley developed MS in 2002 at the tender age of 15 with almost total left-sided paralysis. Due to severe side effects, Conor decided to come off his medications after a couple of months. Instead, he began eating a WFPB diet and has remained symptom-free since. He decided to make a career out of helping people in the same way and has a degree in human nutrition and dietetics as well as a doctorate in nutrition.

Having scoured the scientific evidence around MS for most of his career, he advocates for lifestyles that include moderate sunshine, vitamin D, fruits and veggies, wholegrains, beans and omega-3s. He has found that smoking, stress, salt, animal fat (meat and dairy) and being overweight can negatively impact MS.

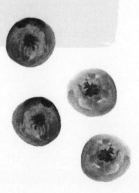

TOP TIPS FOR OPTIMISING IMMUNITY

I have talked broadly about autoimmune conditions, and also about cancer in terms of prevention and lifestyle. But what about infections that we want to minimise and prevent? How do we give our immune system the tools it needs to function well?

A WFPB diet

You guessed it – eat all the colours in fruits and vegetables! A WFPB approach is abundant in antioxidant- and vitamin-rich foods to optimise both your gut bugs and your subsequent immune function.

Boost your sleep

Our T cells and our microbiomes respond directly to the amount of sleep we get – even one day of poor shut-eye can have a big impact. Aim for seven hours minimum every night.

Nasal breathing

It makes sense that nasal hairs and nitric oxide production in the paranasal sinuses are a small but relevant defence to airborne pollution and viruses. Therefore, breathing through the nose can support the body's natural resistance to infection. Nasal breathing also reduces drying out of the airways, which, much like dehydration, can reduce the antibodies in the mucous layer of your respiratory tract. So, drink plenty of water too!

Lymphatic lunges

Get the body moving regularly to allow lymph flow. The movement of your muscles allows lymph fluid to move your immune cells around the body to fight infections.

Vitamin C

When our body is fighting infection, our immune cells use a lot of vitamin C, so it is important to have enough. Vitamin C may shorten the duration of a cold, and it can be found in abundance in oranges, kiwis, peppers and cauliflower to name a few.

Vitamin D

Studies have shown that vitamin D plays an important role in immune response to respiratory pathogens. One study showed that vitamin D deficiency can contribute to poor respiratory functioning and health in middle-aged adults. There is also ongoing research into whether vitamin D supplementation can prevent or treat coronavirus infection.

Zinc

Study data shows zinc can reduce viral replication inside cells, but it is important to get the right amount. It can be obtained from many foods including beans, chickpeas, lentils, tofu, walnuts, flax seeds and wholemeal bread.

Eat more herbs

Fresh crushed garlic (allicin – technically a root) has great antimicrobial effects in several studies; sage, cumin, oregano, thyme, cloves and of course turmeric (curcumin) are all worth adding to your cooking for an extra dose of immune support.

Save yourself from stress

Try to reduce stress or manage it better. Cortisol is an immunosuppressive hormone and to top it all, if you are in an anxious state you are less likely to sleep or eat healthily. This is the hardest tip to follow for some of us, but your body loves you unconditionally and wants you well, so give your body what it needs to help you get there.

I hope you've been able to see the transformative power of a WFPB diet not just in reducing our risk of chronic disease but reversing disease, allowing us to live longer and healthier lives. It has never been so simple to achieve such profound benefits. In the next section, I aim to show you just how easy it is to make the switch and adopt a WFPB lifestyle.

THE SIMPLE SWITCH TO PLANT POWER

'An apple a day keeps the doctor away'.
– Welsh proverb

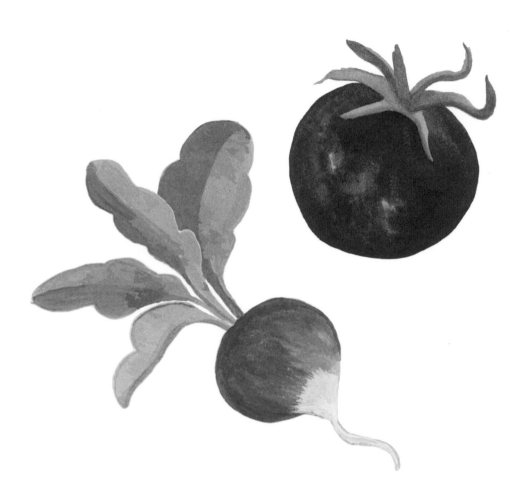

MASTERING THE BUILDING BLOCKS OF WFPB EATING

A wholefoods plant-based diet means a plant-centric diet focusing on wholefoods.

To help you understand what kinds of foods I am referring to, here is a list showing the huge range of things you can eat. Use this to guide your food shopping and remember to eat a rainbow so choose foods of different colours.

WHAT'S INCLUDED IN A WFPB DIET

- **Fruit**
  Bananas, grapes, apples, citrus fruit (grapefruit, lemons, limes, oranges, tangerines), berries (blueberries, blackberries, strawberries, raspberries), avocados, mangoes, peaches, plums, watermelons, melons, papaya, figs, pears, tomatoes, etc.

- **Vegetables**
  Kale, celery, cucumber, onions, spinach, peppers, corn, lettuce, peas, broccoli, turnips, radishes, sweet potatoes, pumpkins, beetroot, parsnips, cauliflower, sprouts, turnips, Swiss chard, lettuce, bok choy, artichokes etc.

- **Wholegrains**
  Wholegrain pasta, bread and cereals, crackers, quinoa, brown rice, oats, barley, wholewheat bread, wholewheat pasta and other starches in their whole form, buckwheat (can be made into noodles), amaranth, teff, millet, popcorn.

- **Nuts and seeds**
  Almonds, Brazil nuts, cashews, hazelnuts, macadamia nuts, pistachio nuts, hazelnuts, pecans, walnuts, hemp seeds, sunflower seeds, chia seeds, sesame seeds, flax seeds, etc.

Beans and legumes

Adzuki beans, chickpeas, black-eyed beans, lentils (red, green, yellow and brown), kidney beans, mung beans, white beans, split peas, peanuts, soya beans, tofu, tempeh, haricot beans, runner beans, broad beans, etc. Some of these foods, such as lentils and chickpeas, can also be made into pasta and flour.

Herbs, spices and seasoning

Oregano, cinnamon, pepper, turmeric, ginger, cardamom, cloves, cacao, coriander, cumin, fennel, nutmeg, paprika, vanilla, basil, lemongrass, mint, oregano, etc. Really, there are too many to list! Condiments such as nutritional yeast, pepper, stock, soy sauce or tamari and liquid smoke are useful too.

Herbs and spices provide flavour and a range of antioxidants to benefit health. Unlike processed sauces that may contain a lot of sugar and salt, herbs and spices can be used liberally and have lots of healthful properties. I love smoked paprika!

Dairy alternatives

Plant milks (such as unsweetened soy, oat, almond, hemp, pea or rice), unsweetened non-dairy yoghurts.

Supplementation:

Vitamin B12 is essential. See the section on supplements (pages 181–84) for further tips. The aim is to get as many nutrients as possible from wholefoods, rather than from supplements.

Plant oils

Many people who have reversed autoimmune issues, improved acne or heart disease symptoms have avoided oil, as we explored in the previous section. This is easy to do once you learn how to water-/stock-fry spices, onion and garlic rather than frying them with oil.

Looking at population studies, most evidence points to the benefits of having poly-unsaturated fats (PUFAs) and mono-unsaturated fats (MUFAs) from plants contributing 20–30 per cent of our diet. You can get both of these fats from eating flax seeds, walnuts and sunflower seeds (PUFA rich foods), and avocados, nut butters and olives (MUFA rich foods). I would advise to prioritise wholefoods like these for the benefits of these healthy plant fats over plant-based oils.

Extra virgin olive oil (EVOO) has been shown to be heart healthy for its MUFAs and the polyphenols it contains. A healthy diet does not require olive oil, but the choice is yours. If you use plant oils, small amounts are needed as they are an energy-dense food.

To see an example of the ideal 'plate', the UK government produced a well-researched 'Eat Well Guide' in 2016 which has been adapted for a plant-based diet by dieticians and researchers from the Plant-based Health Professionals UK in 2019.

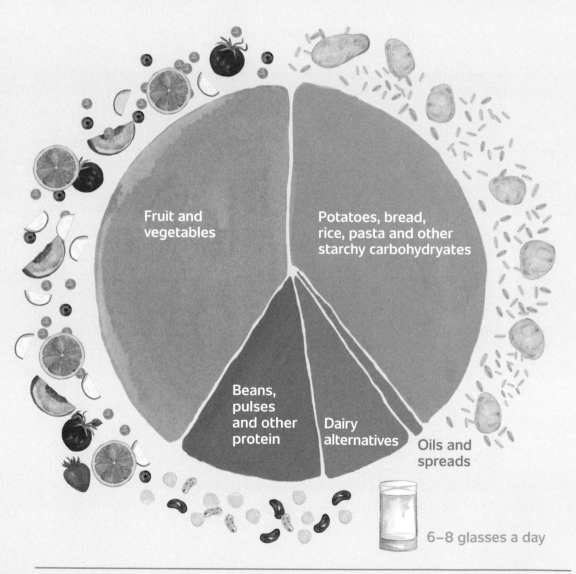

Fruit and vegetables

Potatoes, bread, rice, pasta and other starchy carbohydryates

Beans, pulses and other protein

Dairy alternatives

Oils and spreads

6–8 glasses a day

WHAT'S NOT INCLUDED IN A WFPB DIET

- **Dairy products**

- **Meat**

- **Poultry**

- **Eggs**

- **Fish and seafood**
  All types of fish, including fish sauce.

- **Refined grains**
  White pasta and white bread – wheat that has been heavily milled to remove the bran and germ to give them a finer texture. (Some brown breads are actually white bread coloured with molasses or caramel colouring with seeds added to make them appear to be wholemeal.)

- **Highly processed, high-fat, high-salt and high-sugar foods**
  Fast food, most meat-substitute products (look at the labels – any products with lots of additives and a high-fat, salt and sugar content should be minimised), most shop-bought biscuits, cupcakes, cakes, crisps, pastries etc.

- **Sugary drinks**
  Sugar sweetened fizzy drinks, shop-bought fruit juices, energy drinks, etc.

Many people ask me if it is necessary to go 'all the way' and have a 100 per cent plant-based diet to get all the benefits that I outline in this book. Can we get the same benefits at 80 per cent say, or 90 per cent? I am not aware of any population data that tells us we have to go to 100 per cent for longevity benefits. Plant predominant eating patterns can include Mediterranean, Indian, Thai, Central American, Middle Eastern, African and any number of cuisines. So, the choice is yours. If you have a diagnosis that could be made worse by your food choices, then you might want to go all in with this pattern of eating and see how it makes you feel. Someone who is generally well and just looking for small improvements might choose to use this book to make smaller adjustments – in that case the aim is to maximise the amount of plants they eat for their future health and longevity.

'Everything in moderation' sounds good. But moderation means something different to everyone. And moderation also tends to mean less change is achieved than we want to admit.

One reason why I would encourage you to go all in is for your taste buds. When we put food in our mouths, thousands of taste buds on our tongues, called papillae, sense the chemicals in our food and these attach to receptors, which convey messages to the brain where taste is perceived. These receptors also note the temperature of the food, as well as food that causes a physical sensation, like hot chillies or black pepper. The smell of our food also adds to the flavour as the olfactory receptors in our nose amplify tastes. There is a lot going on!

The good news is that we can overcome the taste-bud hijack by eating less of these products. When we cut out highly processed foods and return to more wholefoods like fruit, veggies, wholegrains and legumes, our taste buds 'reset' and this reset can happen relatively quickly.

Research also shows that the longer you eat a WFPB diet, the more you will enjoy it and the different healthy foods on offer. So, if you can't stand broccoli or hate Brussels sprouts, the key is actually to eat them more often. Cruciferous vegetables are notoriously bitter, however, research has shown that repeated exposure to bitter foods can change the proteins in saliva, making these bitter foods more palatable. Eventually, they will no longer taste bitter. Give it a try!

I wouldn't suggest to a smoker who wants to quit that they smoke one cigarette a day. This may work for some, but I've seen that the best chance of long-lasting change comes with a mindset shift. And when someone does the WFPB approach wholeheartedly, larger benefits can be found. Long-lasting change is also much easier when you have a change in identity. Finding your 'why' and keeping it at the forefront of your mind each day will really help you to feel good about what you are doing. Motivation does not last forever. This is why knowing what you want, feeling good about the little wins and feeling good about yourself is so important.

THE PLANT POWER PLATE

I'm often asked a lot of questions about specific nutrients – exactly how many milligrams of vitamin C and magnesium do I need? What proportions of fats/carbs/protein should I eat with each meal? How many leafy greens should I eat each day? My best advice for you is to relax.

When it comes to numbers, I am reluctant to be too precise for a few reasons. We don't have scientific evidence that fully answers these questions, and the answers depend on how much of each of these nutrients you have in your body already, the integrity of your gut lining, what time of day you ate, what other foods you ate alongside your greens . . . the list goes on.

Virtually nothing in biology is as precise as we would like it to be, but the good news is that eating a varied WFPB diet eliminates the need to worry about all the details. Focus on eating a wide variety of different plant foods and your body will take what it needs and do all the sums for you.

To help you see what proportions of foods a plant power plate would contain, I have taken inspiration from the Canadian Dietary Guidelines, which removed dairy as part of a healthy balanced diet, and prioritised plant sources of protein for health and longevity.

Each day, include half a plate of vegetables or fruit, a quarter plate of plant-based protein, and a quarter plate of wholegrains. In addition, I suggest a side serving of mostly water and occasionally some plant-based milk, to drink. You can see how easily these can all fit into your day in the recipe section (see pages 190–265).

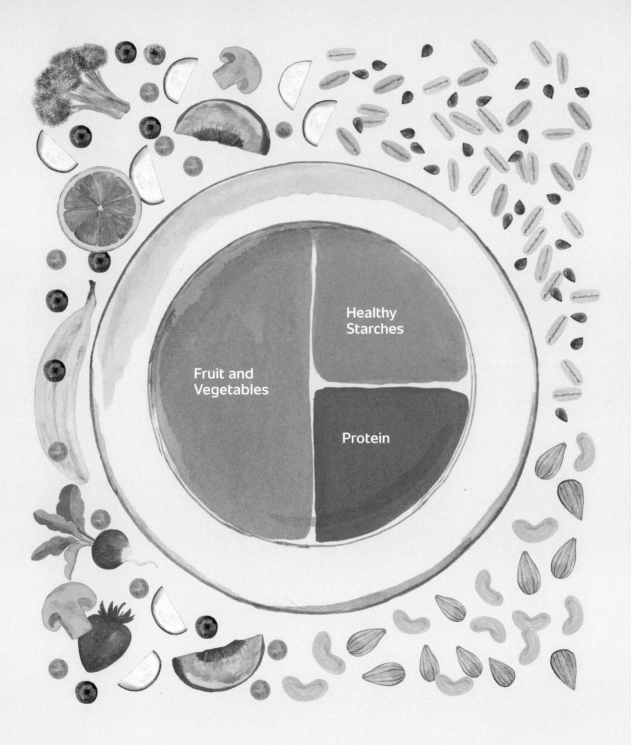

Healthy
Starches

Fruit and
Vegetables

Protein

THE PLANT POWER DOCTOR

Vegetables

Eat as many different types of vegetables as you can, eating as many different colours as possible each day. Aim for cruciferous veggies like broccoli, kale, and cabbage as often as you can too.

Healthy starches

Include starchy vegetables like potatoes, sweet potatoes, butternut squash and pumpkin alongside wholegrains like oatmeal (porridge), quinoa, millet and buckwheat. Starchy foods keep you feeling fuller for longer, and thereby give you more satisfaction too.

Plant-based protein

Many WFPB foods include protein but beans, lentils, chickpeas and peas are especially good, as are nuts and seeds. Soy-containing foods – such as tofu, tempeh and edamame beans – are complete plant proteins containing all amino acids. Choose these ingredients in their least processed states and keep an eye on levels of added salts, sugars and other ingredients.

Fruit

Eat as much as you can in a rainbow of colours. I particularly love berries because they pack the greatest punch when it comes to nutrients.

Water or plant-based milk

It is important to drink lots of fluid every day – at least six to eight glasses – as thirst can be mistaken for hunger. Water is the best option but plant milks and herbal teas also count. While you can get your daily calcium intake from eating WFPB foods, some plant milks are fortified and can help you meet your daily needs. Choose unsweetened fortified varieties if you can. Be mindful of emulsifiers, especially if you have IBD (see pages 122–24).

EATING THE RAINBOW

As we discussed in part 1, fruit and vegetables contain a host of phytochemicals that have a range of positive effects on the body (see page 25). One of the simple ways you can increase the variety of the plants and wholefoods that you eat is to look for lots of colours, textures and shapes. This will help you get all the essential nutrients that you need. Plus, your plate will look pretty good too!

RED: Red peppers, red cabbage, tomatoes, raspberries, watermelon, grapefruit, radishes, rhubarb, red onions, pomegranates, cranberries, cherries, potatoes.

ORANGE: Carrots, sweet potatoes, butternut squash, turmeric root, orange peppers, mangoes, peaches, papaya, satsumas, grapefruit, nectarines, swede.

YELLOW: Sweetcorn, yellow peppers, ginger root, summer squash, lemons.

GREEN: Spinach, kale, broccoli, asparagus, cucumber, avocado, kiwi, green peppers, bok choy, Brussels sprouts, cabbage, celery, green beans, edamame beans, peas, rocket, Swiss chard, okra, apples, mangetout, watercress, leeks.

BLUE/PURPLE: Olives, blueberries, blackberries, plums, aubergines, purple carrots, prunes, raisins.

WHITE: Cauliflower, white beans, garlic, mushrooms, parsnips, seeds, onions, chickpeas, shallots.

EATING 10 A DAY: A DIET OF ABUNDANCE

Many people talk about eating their '5 a day' but is this really the best way to optimal health? While 5 a day is good for you, one large-scale study showed that eating 10 a day could prevent up to 7.8 million premature deaths worldwide every year.

The findings of the 2017 study by Imperial College found that many of us struggle to eat even three or four portions, but research found that eating up to 800g of fruit and vegetables – equivalent to 10 portions and double the recommended amount in the UK – was associated with a 24 per cent reduced risk of heart disease, a 33 per cent reduced risk of stroke, a 28 per cent reduced risk of cardiovascular disease, a 13 per cent reduced risk of total cancer, and a 31 per cent reduction in premature deaths. The bottom line is: the more fruit and veggies we eat, the better!

MAKING SIMPLE SWAPS

Deciding to go for a WFPB diet can be overwhelming for many people to start with. One of the ways I encourage my patients to move towards a plant-focused diet is by making simple swaps. Just think about the meals you usually eat and switch them up for a plant-based alternative.

Most of us tend to eat the same series of meals, maybe even as little as five meals, on rotation. The average is eight to ten. When meat is a key part of our diets it can be hard to imagine a meal that does not contain it, but it's simple if you know how.

If you decide to cook one new thing a week for five weeks, you will have a whole new menu of meals before you know it.

HERE ARE MY TOP SWAPS

- Spaghetti Bolognese ➡ Vegan Bolognese (see page 222)
- Shepherd's Pie ➡ Shepherdless Pie (see page 234)
- Beefburger ➡ Pulled Jackfruit Burger (see page 232)
- Chicken Curry ➡ Vegetable Tikka Masala (see page 238)
- Scrambled Eggs on Toast ➡ Tofu Scramble on Toast (see page 202)
- Lasagne ➡ Veggie Lasagne (see page 223)
- Chilli ➡ Veggie Chilli (see page 221)
- Roast Dinner ➡ Nut and Veggie Roast (see pages 246–47)
- Mac-n-Cheese ➡ Vegan Mac-n-Cheese (made with cashews or soy milk – see page 224)
- Butter ➡ Nut butter
- Mayonnaise ➡ Hummus or cashew-based mayo
- Milk chocolate ➡ Dark chocolate (75% cocoa solids or more)
- Cheese ➡ Nutritional yeast
- Ice cream ➡ Peanut Butter Ice Cream (see page 249)

- Cream ➤ Coconut cream
- Cow's milk ➤ Plant-based milk
- Dairy yoghurt ➤ Soy, almond, cashew or coconut yoghurt
- Sugar and artificial sweeteners ➤ Maple or date syrup

SMART SUPERMARKET CHOICES

I love cooking from scratch, so the food is fresh, made with love and I know exactly what has gone into my meal. But, of course, there are times when we don't have the time or inclination to cook. When someone asks me if home cooked is always better than store bought, I will often say 'it depends'. I had one patient, an elderly gentleman, who had never cooked and did not want to cook, so I suggested he buy a plant-based ready meal at his nearest supermarket. The results were incredible.

He had Type 2 diabetes and had oral medication as well as injectable insulin to attempt to control it. Unfortunately, he was struggling, and his blood sugars were all over the place. Once he started eating the WFPB ready meals, his insulin needs dropped so dramatically he had to cut his insulin in half within three days. He worried this meant he was getting more unwell. I explained the good news, that his new food choices were making him more insulin sensitive and that he needed less medication! After a week of close monitoring he was able to drop his insulin needs by two-thirds, and by the end of a month had come off it entirely, all using ready meals. It would be better if he was cooking for himself, but he couldn't.

These meals were healthier than his previous diet and got him into a far better place health-wise. He then began to make some basic recipes at home, inspired by how much better he felt. This enabled him to up his plant intake even more and reap further benefits from cooking with fresh wholefood ingredients. Often the first step towards health can be the hardest, but it can be the beginning of an amazing journey to a healthier you.

If cooking from scratch is too much for your right now, that's OK. I love to see my patients do whatever works, because it is more likely to stick.

MY TOP TIPS FOR SUPERMARKET SHOPPING

Check the labels when you go shopping, and make a note of the foods that you like the best so that you can shop quicker next time. Choose foods that carry a green or amber label, and avoid any red labels as they are high in saturated fat and sugar. If you're able to shop online, you can find the nutritional information listed on the product page.

- Reduced and low fat are not the same. Low fat means a product has 3g or less fat per 100g, while reduced fat means a product is 25 per cent lower in fat than the standard product. Often reduced-fat products were very high in fat to start with, so the reduced-fat version is still likely to be high in fat.

- Sugar is not always listed as sugar – it can sometimes be called sucrose, glucose, palm sugar, hydrolysed starch, fructose, maltose, honey, syrup and invert sugar. The higher up on the ingredients list sugar is, the more added sugar is in the product.

- If products are listed as 'sugar-free', check for fats that may have replaced the sugars. If products are listed as 'fat free', check for sugars that may have replaced the fats!

- If you are choosing between two similar products, check out the fibre content. If one has more fibre, choose that, so you eat more fibre as part of your daily diet.

WFPB ON A BUDGET

When many people think about a WFPB shopping list they may be concerned about the cost.

It is true that certain supplements and ingredients can be costly, especially meat and dairy replacements, like artisanal nut cheeses. However, the foods that form the backbone of the longest-lived cultures in the world – fruit, veg, rice and beans – are some of the cheapest foods available.

The great thing about whole, unprocessed foods is that they are almost guaranteed to be the cheapest ingredients in the shop! The majority of meals can be made with foods that you already have in your cupboards and a WFPB diet can be tailored to any income.

Here are some ways to save money when shopping and cooking:

Buy in bulk

It may sound obvious, but if you have the space, buy foods that you use a lot and that have a long shelf life in bulk. For example, nuts, grains, dried legumes and herbs and spices will all have long dates on them. Look for the unit price on the shelf with the product description, which will tell you the cost per weight. This makes it easy to compare products to choose the cheapest ones.

Buy dry

Beans and legumes in tins and cartons are always cheaper than meat (and it pays to stock up when they are on offer) but dried beans and lentils are even cheaper and will yield double their weight when cooked. If you like the convenience of cooked beans and have space in your freezer, you can always cook a bulk load and then freeze them in portions.

Make it yourself

Where you can, cook from scratch. It is always cheaper and often very easy once you know how. Make a plan for the week and set aside a few hours to cook a large batch of meals and make good use of your freezer space. Buy some reusable containers and freeze in portions. Then all you need to do is get them out, defrost and heat up, like a ready meal.

Leftovers for lunch

If you make an evening meal and do not want to batch cook, make a little extra, so you can eat it for lunch the next day. This is a great habit to get into because shop-bought lunches can get expensive. Regular surveys often conclude that you can save well over £1,000 a year by doing this. Even taking snacks from home will save you money and will usually be a healthier and more nutritious choice.

Buy frozen

Frozen fruit and veggies are extremely convenient and often cheaper than fresh versions. They are usually packed ripe and frozen straight away, so they will be full of nutritional value. Sometimes they have even more nutrients than fresh foods. If you know you are not going to eat your vegetables within a day or two, this is often the better option.

Buy in season and at the right quantities

Seasonal produce not only tastes better but will often be cheaper. Ensure you choose just the right quantities of fresh foods as these go off quickly, so only buy what you know you will eat to avoid food waste.

Get savvy with vegan products

Vegan products can be expensive and heavily processed and sometimes not as healthy. Check the labels for ingredients, salt and sugar.

Make lists but adapt them

One of the great things about a WFPB diet is how flexible and adaptable recipes can be. When you hit the shops, take a list but you do not need to stick to it too rigidly. For example, if you are planning to buy peaches and there is an offer on plums, buy those instead. Does the broccoli looks like it is on the turn? Use cauliflower, kale or cabbage.

Shop around and look down

Supermarket-own brands will often match the quality of big brands but at a much lower cost. Sometimes, you will find the lower-priced items on the bottom shelves; the most expensive are often placed at eye level. Asian stores can also be a great place to buy tofu, tempeh, miso, spice mixes, soy sauce, coconut milk and other items at fantastic prices. And search Turkish or Indian stores for herbs, spices and fresh vegetables as well as items like dates, nuts and dried legumes for a fraction of the price.

Shop at local markets

It is often easier to do all your shopping at the supermarket, but if you have the time it can pay to shop around. Once you are a seasoned pro, shopping at local markets is a good way to pick up local produce at the most affordable prices. Local markets often stock cheap fruit and vegetables from local suppliers, so you are also supporting them. Go early for the biggest selections and towards the end of the day for special offers.

Choose local veg boxes

I am a big fan of local vegetable boxes because they support local farmers. These can be inexpensive and typically have less packaging and more organic options.

IS ORGANIC PRODUCE IMPORTANT?

Is organic food really worth the higher price of conventionally grown foods? After all, peer-reviewed science lacks strong evidence that organic produce is more nutritious than conventionally farmed foods. The truth is, all food used to be organic. With the advent of the first insecticide in 1939, DDT was used by the American military to great effect in killing off the lice, mosquitoes and fleas that spread malaria and typhus. Then a farming revolution began, which saw crops that were once ravaged by insects protected with ease. However, DDT was banned in the UK in 1986 when it was discovered to be harmful to wildlife and the environment. It can persist in the soil for up to 15 years and is still used globally in countries such as India and China. Many other types of insecticide are still in use across the globe today.

It is hard to assess the effect of these insecticides across a human lifespan. There is no doubt that even insecticides deemed safe for humans will harm our microbiome – they are, after all, designed to kill bugs. Some research has linked pesticide exposure to allergies in children and Alzheimer's in the elderly. There is little doubt that glyphosate-based herbicides are linked to the development of non-Hodgkin's lymphoma as well. In a large study from 2018 of more than 68,000 French volunteers, people who ate organic food were found to have a lower overall risk of cancer.

That being said, not all studies point in this direction, and it is important to remember that almost all the population studies we have on how beneficial fruits and vegetables are come from data on people eating conventionally grown foods.

The bottom line for health is this – the best fruits and vegetables you can eat are the ones you can afford. Cost should not prevent you from eating these healthy foods. It is always better to eat more fruits and vegetables, wherever they come from.

What about environmental concerns? Bees play a significant role in the pollination of the foods that we eat. As bee populations die from the overuse of pesticides, this has a dramatic effect on the way our food is pollinated. In parts of China, the native bee population is so low that farmers have to 'hand' pollinate their crops. Scientists are now creating pollination drones in case bees can no longer pollinate our fruit. But it is not just the bees – the effects on the soil of chemical-heavy farming and tillage is just as much of a problem.

Soil erosion means topsoil is washed away into the ocean with heavy rainfall, rather than absorbing the rain water into the soil. This puts our ability to grow food at risk. So we have to act now.

What is the solution? Conservation agricultural methods. These minimise tillage (mechanical soil disturbance) and allow cover crops to protect the soil. This has a number of benefits. It allows earthworms to live undisturbed; breaking down dead plant materials and creating humus, a natural fertiliser. It also allows underground fungal networks (mycorrhiza) to connect individual plants, allowing them to transfer water, carbon, nitrogen and other nutrients and minerals to each other. Maintaining this soil structure allows life and nutrients back to our soils. All of this is destroyed by tillage. Conservation agriculture often goes hand in hand with organic practices too, but not always.

Farmers are agricultural superheroes. They work incredibly hard to provide our food, under increasing pressure and narrowing margins. We need to be grateful for them and show our support. When farmers are passionate about shifting towards a healthier way to work with the soil, and when governments support them, we will be on our way to a more sustainable and self-reliant food system.

But what if you're just one person living life and eating these foods? What can you do? Buying more plant-based options will be absolutely vital. Scientific data shows that an economy heavily reliant on a meat, dairy and fisheries industries is unsustainable for the planet. *Science* journal published a ground-breaking study in 2018 investigating how to achieve sustainable animal agriculture. The study analysed over 40,000 farms in nearly 120 countries and concluded that it just wasn't possible to sustain the farming of animals for food. Plastics pollution, the death of insect populations and the destruction of habitats also mean our children will have to face some hard choices unless we take action now.

What can we do? Eat a more plant-based diet. Support local farmers who are using conservation techniques to grow food. If you don't have anyone locally doing that, buying organic if you can afford to could be a step in the right direction. Maybe even grow your own if you can – this is hard work and will give you even more gratitude for our farmers.

During the Second World War, there was a 'dig for victory' government campaign that captured the imagination of millions of people, who saw it as a way to contribute to the war effort. This 'garden front' was hugely important for alleviating food shortages and by 1942 half the UK population was part of the effort to create vegetable patches wherever they could. There was an explosion in the use of allotments, and even the moat of the Tower of London was used to grow vegetables! The US had a similar campaign, the 'Victory Gardens', and by 1943, 40 per cent of all vegetables eaten in the US was grown in these garden plots. We may never return to that. But in an age where topsoil erosion, land-mass degradation and global pandemics have the power to disrupt food supplies, growing locally and seasonally has never been more important.

HOW TO KEEP WFPB FUN

One of the main stumbling blocks so many people have is that they are not confident with cooking. But don't worry, with a bit of creativity and some recipes ideas (see pages 190–265), you can have a plate bursting with nutrients, taste and variety.

Sometimes we all get stuck in food 'ruts' where we struggle to feel excited by the food on our plates. We figure out our 'go-to' meals and then eat them over (and over) again. Maybe it's toast for breakfast, followed by the same sandwich for lunch and one of a small handful of evening meals.

Here are some ideas to help you break out of these cycles:

- **Try new herbs and spices**
  The right herb can transform your meal, adding new depth, colour and aroma. Herbs and spices are often spoken of in the same breath but they are different. Spices are aromatic seasonings that come from the roots, buds, bark, seeds, fruit, and berries of different plants and trees. Common ones include cinnamon (which comes from bark), peppercorns from berries and paprika from the fruit of a plant. Herbs mainly come from plant leaves and the most common ones include basil, oregano, rosemary, thyme, parsley, sage and chives. Turmeric and black pepper, for example, are a particularly powerful combination because they increase the amount of curcumin, known to reduce inflammation, which can be absorbed by the body (known as bioavailability) by up to 2,000 per cent. I've added some details about my favourite medicinal herbs and their uses on pages 158–59.

Switch your grains

We all love rice and this can form the staple of many meals but there are countless other grains that can blend seamlessly with dishes too, including oats, quinoa, amaranth, barley, buckwheat, couscous, millet, farro, teff, spelt and wheat berries. Before I went plant-based I'd never heard of some of these – a foreign language of new and fancy grains! Brown rice, wholemeal pasta and quinoa are my absolute favourites but I also really like buckwheat noodles and penne pasta made from lentil, edamame or chickpea flour for a combo of protein and fibre!

Head down a new aisle

Next time you head to the shops, aim to put one new veggie in your basket and cook something with it. This is why veg boxes are so great as they push you into trying something original. You're bound to discover something out-of-the-ordinary, which you love.

Go international

Try to incorporate ideas from around the world in your diet. For example, a tofu scramble could be made with black beans and chilli-based spices to have a Mexican twist, or add ginger, sesame and peanut to a dish for a Chinese flavour. Harissa paste and dried fruits could add a Moroccan feel. Garam masala is one of my favourite Indian spice mixes to make a meal more delicious!

Asian
Cinnamon, cloves, star anise, fennel, peppercorns.

Indian
Coriander, cumin, mustard seeds, turmeric, fenugreek, ginger, chilli, onion, garlic, cardamom, cloves, bay leaf.

Italian
Basil, rosemary, thyme, oregano, parsley, garlic.

Mexican
Basil, chilli, cumin, onion, coriander.

Thai
Chilli, lemongrass, garlic, coriander, Thai basil.

Jerk
Chilli, thyme, coriander, cinnamon, ginger, cloves, garlic, onions.

MEDICINAL HERBS

Many medications I rely on to treat my patients have their roots in nature: aspirin is from willow bark, digoxin is extracted from foxgloves and morphine is derived from poppies. The herbal remedies I mention below are not regulated in the same way as pharmaceuticals, and have not been investigated and distilled for widespread therapeutic use. But this does not negate the fact that they can have effects on the human body worth understanding. It is always a good policy to look for a registered herbal medicine, with the THR logo on the pack, to ensure you are getting a quality product independently assessed. So, with that in mind, here are my top herbs that you may wish to add to your self-care toolbox.

- **Aloe vera**
  Used for the treatment and soothing of burns for many years, this plant has also been found to have antimicrobial properties and potential benefits in the management of diabetes and ulcerative colitis.

- **Amla**
  Also known as Indian gooseberry, this adaptogenic herb can balance your immune system, and a double blind randomised controlled trial showed a twice daily dosage of 500mg could also reduce cholesterol and triglycerides in patients with high blood lipids. It has been found to have a variety of benefits in pre-clinical trials including liver protective and anti-diabetic effects.

- **Ashwaghandha**
  Also known as Indian ginseng, this herb has been used in Ayurveda for boosting vitality and mood, while several studies show benefits for reducing anxiety, and one interesting trial showed improved hormone levels in men (DHEA and testosterone), which may explain the reported benefits of ashwaghanda for treating fatigue.

- **Berberine**
  This is a compound that can be extracted from several plants, and is most commonly taken by mouth for diabetes, high levels of cholesterol or other fats in the blood (hyperlipidemia), and high blood pressure. It has a variety of ways of reducing inflammatory pathways in the body and animal trials have shown benefits for reducing the severity of heart attacks and heart failure.

Boswellia

Also known as Indian frankincense, this herb is used to reduce inflammation and can be an effective painkiller.

Neem

This is a herb with antibacterial, anti-parasitic and anti-fungal properties and has also been found to be useful for people with dry, itchy, red skin conditions.

Mushrooms

There are a whole range of beautiful mushrooms with general health benefits, in part due to their beta-glucans content. Much like oats, these soluble fibres help improve cholesterol, heart health and blood sugars. Notable among them is reishi, which has been nicknamed 'the mushroom of immortality' due to its immune-system-protecting polysaccharides, and has been shown more generally to reduce inflammation and calm the mind. Lion's mane is said to be beneficial for brain health, cordyceps for exercise performance, and turkey tail and chaga for immune-system regulation, among other things.

Sigisbeckia

This traditional Chinese herb is used for the relief of arthritis, back ache, joint and muscle pain. Pre-clinical trials show reduced inflammation to the cartilage within joints with similar modes of action to anti-inflammatory painkillers (without reported gastrointestinal side effects).

Turmeric

Used as a medicinal spice for 4,000 years, it has multiple potential benefits primarily due to its anti-inflammatory and antioxidant effects. It has been shown to benefit metabolic syndrome, provide pain relief, and is also helpful in the management of inflammatory and degenerative conditions. Always pair it with black pepper as the piperine in it allows for proper absorption of this distinctive golden spice.

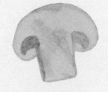
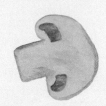

DAIRY: YES OR NO?

The big question about dairy: yes or no? Many people have made their minds up about this, with some firmly in the 'yes' camp and some rooted in the 'no' camp. Milk is a good source of calcium. But is it really necessary?

You see, although dairy is a useful source of calcium and nutrients, especially in times of scarcity, there is no biological reason why humans require milk from another species after weaning. Humans have adapted to drinking cow's milk after we started domesticating animals, especially in northern Europe. The enzyme lactase is needed to break down the milk sugar lactose. Adults' ability to digest the lactose in cow's milk is called 'lactase persistence' – most people do not have this ability after they are babies. A large study published in 2017 shows that the global prevalence of lactose intolerance due to lack of lactase activity is 68 per cent, and in those affected, consuming dairy products leads to diarrhoea, bloating, cramps, nausea or headaches.

Along with yoghurt and cheese, cow's milk is a source of amino acids, riboflavin, phosphorus and calcium. However, dairy's place in a balanced diet is increasingly being questioned, partly because of intensive farming practices and the environmental cost of the dairy industry but the health benefits are also now being re-evaluated.

A compilation of studies found no correlation between drinking more milk and lowering risk of bone fracture. In fact, some studies show that fracture rates and premature mortality are highest in populations with the greatest milk consumption. While milk can contribute to nutrition, it is noted that galactose, a sugar found in milk, has been shown to induce oxidative stress and chronic inflammation (see pages 26–30). These chronic inflammatory states are associated with heart disease, cancer, bone and muscle loss.

Dairy has been associated with increased rates of prostate, breast and ovarian cancer in some population studies. Colorectal cancer rates appear lower with dairy consumption, but other serious bowel conditions could be exacerbated by it. For example, scientists have found a bacterium contained in milk, mycobacterium avium paratuberculosis (MAP), which releases a molecule that prevents our blood cells from killing E. coli, a bacterium known to be in high numbers in Crohn's disease bowel tissue. This same bacterium has also been implicated in the development of Type 1 diabetes. There is also evidence emerging that links rheumatoid arthritis to MAP exposure in those who are genetically susceptible. Small amounts of MAP survive the pasteurisation process, and traces of it can also be contained in the meat from a cow.

There are some parts of the world where people rely on dairy for important nutrition, especially where resources are scarce. But overall it is clear there are also downsides to dairy. The recent Canadian Dietary Guidelines have removed dairy products completely from their recommendations, and many people are turning away from dairy for environmental reasons too.

HOW MUCH CALCIUM DO I NEED?

Calcium is the most abundant mineral in our bodies. It is found in the ground, which is why plants are an excellent source of calcium. Calcium is crucial for healthy bones and teeth, but it also plays other important roles, such as regulating metabolism, for muscle function, proper blood flow, nerve transmission and the release of hormones. About 99 per cent of our calcium is stored in the body's bones and teeth.

The recommended daily calcium intake in the UK is:

- Adults aged 19 to 64 years: 700mg
- Children aged 11 to 18 years: 800–1,000mg
- Children aged 7 to 10 years: 550mg
- Children aged 4 to 6 years: 450mg
- Children aged 1 to 3 years: 350mg

A large number of people do not meet these recommendations. Breastfeeding mums, post-menopausal women and people with coeliac disease or inflammatory bowel conditions, for example, may need slightly more.

Many people also smoke, or drink a lot of caffeine and alcohol, which can interfere with the way the body absorbs calcium. A high salt intake can also have an impact.

Our bodies do an amazing job of carefully regulating the amount of calcium that is in our bloodstream, so it doesn't change according to our dietary intake. If we do not get enough calcium from our diets to 'top up' the reservoir, the body takes the calcium from the bones to ensure normal cell function. This can lead to weakened bones, called osteoporosis, a heightened risk of fractures and broken bones.

Most fruits and vegetables have been shown to increase bone density and bone health. Some vegetables contain oxalates, an organic compound that can bind to calcium in your gut, making it hard for your body to absorb it. Studies have shown that the body may only absorb 5 per cent of calcium found in high-oxalate vegetables, such as spinach, rhubarb and Swiss chard. Boiling these veg reduces oxalate levels by 30 to 80 per cent (and is more effective than steaming or baking) although it also diminishes nutrients like vitamin C. Cruciferous vegetables – e.g. kale, okra, Brussels sprouts and broccoli – are rich in calcium and low in oxalate. We can absorb lots of calcium from these veggies, and they have many other health benefits too.

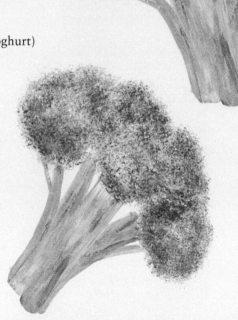

Plant sources of calcium include:

- Calcium-fortified plant milks, cereals and juices
- Calcium-set tofu
- Other soy-based foods (tempeh, tofu, yoghurt)
- Collard greens
- Bok choi
- Kale
- Broccoli
- Cauliflower
- Cabbage
- Tahini
- Watercress
- Beans
- Peas
- Lentils
- Nuts including Brazil nuts, almonds, walnuts, pistachio nuts, hazelnuts and macadamia nuts, as well as nut butters like almond butter.

- Seeds, such as chia and sesame seeds.

- Seaweed

- Fresh and dried fruits like figs, dried apricots and prunes.

CALCIUM AND VITAMIN D

In order for calcium to be absorbed by the intestines, vitamin D must be present. Sunlight is the main source of vitamin D – we make around 90 per cent of our vitamin D through our skin. In winter, when the days are shorter, vitamin D deficiency can be a problem depending on the amount of pigment in our skin. I recommend taking a daily supplement in winter months to anyone, and throughout the year if you are unable to regularly get outdoors. The remaining 10 per cent of our vitamin D comes from food. Fatty fish, liver and egg yolks are concentrated vitamin D sources. On a WFPB diet, good plant sources of vitamin D include mushrooms, fortified plant milks, cereals and tofu.

PLANT MILKS: WHICH ARE THE BEST?

The most environmentally friendly plant milks to produce are oat and soy milks. Rice milk and almond milk require a lot of water to make, although still half the amount of water required to make the equivalent amount of cow's milk. All these plant milks produce just a third of the greenhouse gases made in the production of cow's milk, and ten times less land is required to produce the equivalent quantity of plant milk to cow's milk. Some food for thought. But what about taste? Which plant milk will be best for your latte or to make a creamy sauce?

- **Oat milk**
  Made by soaking and blending whole oats in water, oat milk has a creamy texture and lots of fibre. Many brands are fortified with additional vitamins and minerals, such as calcium, iodine and vitamin D. It is also excellent for added fibre and is a great choice for reducing environmental impact. It's delicious on cereal, creamy in cooking and in tea and coffee.

- **Soy milk**
  This is made by soaking soya beans that are ground into a liquid and boiled. It is most nutritionally similar to cow's milk and is a good source of protein and calcium and often fortified with additional vitamins and minerals. Soy milk has a similar consistency to cow's milk so is popular for using on cereal,

adding to your cuppa, or for cooking and baking. This is my favourite milk and ideal for porridge and using in coffee and tea.

Coconut milk

This is different to the tinned version of coconut milk because it is made using blended grated coconut in hot water and separating the water content. It can have a high-fat content and tends to have a higher sugar content than other plant-based milks. Coconut milk is excellent for cooking and baking.

Almond milk

Made like oat milk, by soaking and blending whole almonds in water, it is high in vitamin E, which is important for skin health and immunity. This is also a popular choice over breakfast cereals and with porridge because it has a creamy and nutty texture. It is lower in protein than soy and oat milk.

Cashew milk

This is made like almond milk using cashew nuts and is also rich in vitamin E and contains fewer calories. It is also often fortified with additional vitamins, like vitamin D. It is great in coffee and lattes because of its thick texture.

Hazelnut milk

Hazelnuts are roasted, soaked and blended with water to create this rich-flavoured milk. It is naturally high in calcium and folate and popular for cooking or adding to tea and coffee.

Pea milk

Made by grounding yellow split peas into a flour and then separating the starch and protein and mixing with water, pea milk has a similar taste to other plant-based milks. It is a great protein source and some are supplemented with DHA, a key omega-3 fatty acid.

Hemp milk

Made by blending the seeds of a hemp plant with water, hemp milk is a good source of calcium and omega-3 and omega-6 fatty acids and is low in saturated fat. It has a thin texture and nutty taste, so it goes better with granola or porridge. It is an allergen-friendly milk for kids and suitable for toddlers. If making homemade nut milk, you can add ¼ cup of hemp seeds to boost the nutrient and protein content.

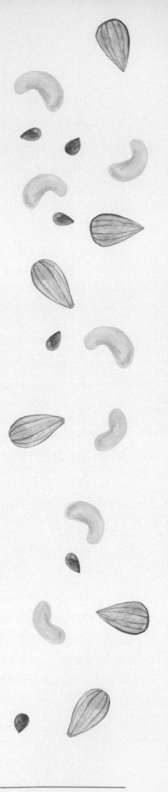

- **Rice milk**

  Made from milled rice and water, rice milk is naturally sweet, contains no saturated fat and is low in calories. However, it is not a good source of protein or calcium unless it has been fortified. It often has added sugars too, so watch out for these.

PLANT PROTEIN

Proteins are the building blocks of life. These large, complex molecules play many important roles and are required for the structure, function, and regulation of our tissues and organs. They are essential for a number of key bodily functions, including blood clotting, immune-system response and hormone production. Proteins are made up of many amino acids connected in a chain. When we eat, our bodies break down these proteins into amino acid blocks with different sequences, depending on what types of protein we need. Shorter chains of amino acids are called peptides.

Certain amino acids that we eat are essential and there are nine that our body does not make, so we must eat them. Proteins containing an abundance of all nine of these essential proteins are called complete. Meat is a complete protein. You may hear some nutritional advisors tell you that plant proteins are not complete. They may also say strict food combining is needed in order to get enough protein from plants. Neither of these things is true. Complete proteins are found in quinoa, tofu, tempeh, edamame, amaranth, buckwheat and hemp seeds for example.

You do not have to think about actively combining plants in order to obtain enough protein. Our bodies cycle amino acids over a roughly 48-hour period, so they really do not need to all be eaten at once. As long as you get a variety of complementary proteins over the course of a day, you will always get ample sources of every amino acid. This is very easy to do. On a chemical level, by the time you have eaten and absorbed the amino acids, it makes no difference whether they have come from animal or plant sources.

Kwashiorkor is the medical name for protein deficiency and is an extremely rare condition that occurs in states of famine. Never heard of it? Most people haven't. For most people, a protein deficiency is not something to worry about.

HOW MUCH PROTEIN DO WE REALLY NEED?

Bariatric surgeon Garth Davis, M.D. wrote eloquently in his book *Proteinaholic* that if we in the Western world spent half as much time worrying about whether we had had enough fibre as we do about whether we have enough protein, we'd be far healthier as a society.

We need much less protein than we think. Our protein requirements are dictated by our activity levels and weight. Most adults need around 0.75g of protein per kilogram of body weight per day. For the average woman, this is 45g and for the average man is 55g. That's about a cup of cooked lentils and a cup of tofu per day. As a guide, a protein portion should fit into the palm of your hand (and take up no more than a quarter of your plate, see page 146).

Although protein is essential, it is important to understand we can sometimes get too much of a good thing. There is much published data on protein being associated with cellular ageing, and animal proteins specifically being associated with higher mortality rates. Kidney disease patients will do badly on the so-called 'meat-sweet' diet. A 2018 review of 17 studies reported that a very low protein intake seems to slow the progression of kidney failure. Animal proteins cause a phenomenon called 'hyperfiltration', which results in an increase in the workload of the kidney. This isn't harmful if it only happens occasionally, but if we are eating animal proteins for most meals every day, especially with impaired kidneys, it becomes hard work. This hyper-filtration process happens quickly – eat some tuna and within three hours your kidney filtration rate can shoot up by 36 per cent. Meat-based diets are largely acid-producing and can cause metabolic problems for those with impaired kidney function.

Plants rich in protein are also rich in fibre and phytochemicals, and low in saturated fat, as well as containing no cholesterol. All these factors are linked to a lower risk of chronic diseases and early death. Animal proteins contain some micronutrients, but they also come with a side serving of saturated fat, cholesterol, antibiotics (in non-organic animal products) and other inflammatory compounds.

It makes more sense to me that we eat plant proteins and absorb all their many benefits directly, rather than feed them to animals so we can eat animal protein without the phytochemical benefits and with these unnecessary added extras.

My hope is that patients with kidney disease will soon be offered the chance to understand the benefits of a WFPB diet when the guidelines catch up with the research on this important issue. When longevity research also suggests that having a diet too high in protein is associated with reduced lifespan, it is certainly time to rethink our protein obsession and remember that real plant foods contain all the protein we could ever need.

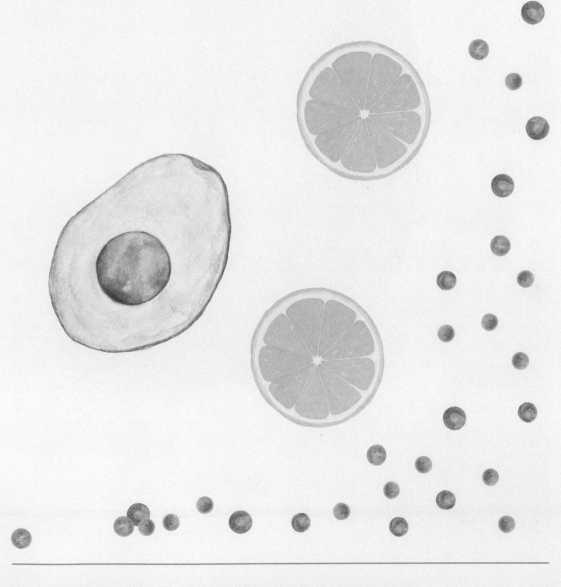

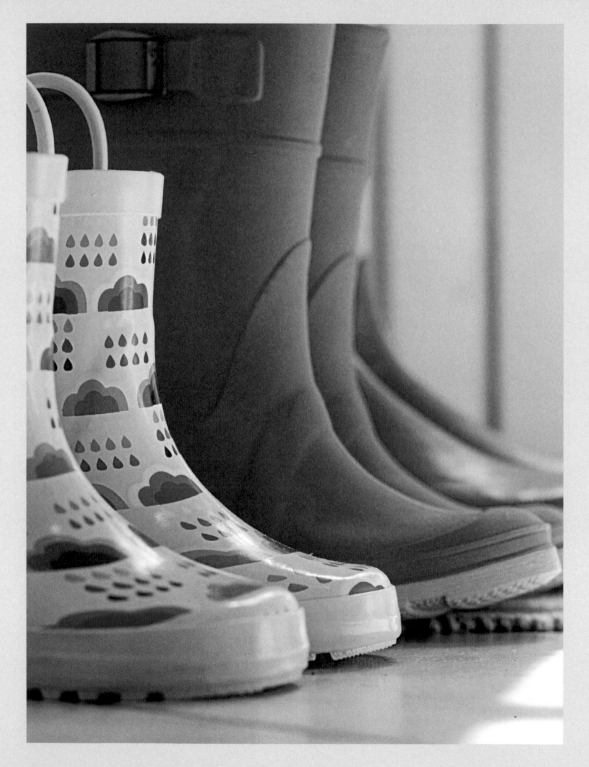

THE PLANT POWER DOCTOR

WFPB FOR FAMILIES

One of the questions I am asked most is whether a WFPB diet is suitable for children, pregnant women and elderly people. The answer is yes! People may have different priorities depending on their age and fitness, but the health benefits of a well-planned plant-based lifestyle are available to anyone at any age. A WFPB diet has been deemed suitable for all stages of life by the Academy of Nutrition and Dietetics (formerly the American Dietetic Association) and the British Dietetic Association.

As an 82-year-old patient of mine once said to me, 'It is never too late to make the switch'. He used a WFPB approach to finally get his blood pressure under control after years of tinkering with medications with little success.

Let's look at the important stages of life and what you need to know for each one. I am hoping this will be a helpful roadmap, not just for you but also for those that you love.

PREGNANCY

Creating new life is one of life's greatest gifts. Everyone's circumstances are different; a baby may be dearly longed for or a complete surprise, which may bring with it some uncertainty or even anxiety. But everyone has two things in common: they want their baby to grow healthily, and they want to have a happy and healthy pregnancy. Although a WFPB pregnancy offers very real advantages for the health of mum and baby, this does not give a free pass to chow down on vegan ice cream, cookies and cakes – pregnancy cravings aside!

Having a baby can be an overwhelming time, so don't be too hard on yourself in pursuit of drastic changes. That being said, it is good to think about optimising your pregnancy health of course, and what better time to do so?

When you know you are pregnant, you must tell your family doctor and get your maternity healthcare arranged. You will need to discuss your medical history and if you have any pre-existing medical conditions, it's important to ask your doctor for advice.

It is a widespread misconception that you need to eat double the amount of calories during pregnancy. Your calorie needs will only increase modestly – it is recommended by the NHS that pregnant women should only eat an extra 200 calories in the last three months of their pregnancy. But your nutrient needs will increase during pregnancy – you will require more protein and more folic acid, for example. Maximise fruit, veggies, pulses and wholegrains that are rich in these nutrients. If you suffer from morning sickness, you may tolerate soups, stews and ice-cold smoothies over raw vegetables and salads.

Existing research indicates that a well-planned plant-based diet rich in fibre and micronutrients and low in saturated fat is likely to be protective against medical conditions in pregnancy such as pre-eclampsia, gestational diabetes and preterm delivery.

It is vital to take a prenatal vitamin supplement to ensure a baseline level of vitamins for your growing baby, ideally from the time you begin trying for a baby. This advice applies to all women, whatever their pre-existing health and eating habits. Check the supplement contains a few key nutrients, which will also be important after delivery and with breastfeeding. Iron supplementation is essential to prevent and treat iron deficiency anaemia. Folic acid (at least 400mcg/day) from a mixture of foods and supplements is needed to avoid neural tube defects like spina bifida. In addition, adequate levels of vitamin D (600UI/day), choline (450mg/day), iodine (220mcg/day) and calcium (1,200mg/day) are needed for the normal growth and brain development of your baby.

OK, now let's take a more detailed look at important nutrients and where to find them:

- **Protein**
  Protein is crucial to help grow a healthy baby. Pregnant women should aim for about 70g protein per day during the second and third trimesters to support fluid and tissue production. It's easy to meet this requirement by eating a variety of plant-based foods. High-protein options include lentils, beans, tofu, seeds, quinoa, chickpeas and nut butters.

- **Calcium**
  Calcium is very important for the development of your baby's bones and teeth, especially during the third trimester, and can

be found in abundance in kale, bok choy, lettuce, cabbage, figs, beans, sesame seeds, tahini, almonds, almond butter, chia seeds, beans, edamame, tofu and fortified plant milks, cereals and juices.

Vitamin D

The natural source of vitamin D is sunlight. If you do not get regular sunlight, vitamin D is also available in vitamins and in fortified foods such as plant milks, cereals and mushrooms. I'd still suggest a supplement.

Vitamin B12

Vitamin B12 can also be found in fortified foods like Marmite, nutritional yeast, cereals and fortified plant milks. We only need small amounts but as it is essential for development of your baby's nervous system and brain it's always worth taking a supplement. It can be found in all standard multivitamins and in prenatal vitamins. I'd recommend taking at least 10mcg daily of vitamin B12 if you are eating a WFPB diet, or if you decide to take a weekly supplement go for a 2,000mcg dose. (See the supplements section for more information on vitamin B12.)

Iron

Many women get low in iron during pregnancy. This is in part because blood volume increases by around 50 per cent so there is a dilution effect, with more blood fluid carrying the same amount of red blood cells. But iron needs are still double what they would normally be (27mg from 15mg). So, make sure you are eating plenty of lentils, chickpeas, beans, tofu, dried fruits and cashews. Enjoying leafy greens like kale, spinach, rocket and other salad leaves that provide a rich source of vitamin C to aid absorption will be important too. Some people still end up unable to meet their iron requirements whatever their diet and will need a supplement temporarily. Don't neglect to check this and make sure you are getting enough, as it can affect the baby's birth weight and cause preterm delivery if you are anaemic. If you do need an iron supplement, make sure you drink plenty of water, get your body moving and get your fibre from fruit and veggies to help prevent constipation! Take your supplement in between meals (especially those containing legumes like lentils and green beans) and not with tea or coffee, so that you optimise your iron absorption.

Iodine

Iodine is the forgotten element and is essential in the human body for the production of thyroid hormones (see pages 109–10). When a developing baby is deprived of iodine, it can result in congenital hypothyroidism. This is a serious problem, which can cause mental retardation and growth problems. Current recommendations for daily iodine doses are 250mcg for pregnant and breastfeeding women. The most reliable way to know you have enough is with a supplement, particularly if you are pregnant or breastfeeding. Selenium is important too, so we can absorb just the right amount of iodine. Great plant-based sources include Brazil nuts, mushrooms, beans and sunflower seeds.

Omega-3 fatty acids

These are essential fats and they come in three forms; ALA, EPA and DHA. Alpha-linolenic acid (or ALA) comes from plants and EPA/DHA comes from algae and fish primarily. UK NHS guidelines advise pregnant women to limit oily fish to no more than two portions a week to limit the baby's exposure to heavy metals. Luckily, we can convert plant-sourced ALA into EPA and DHA. This process is made more efficient if we have a good balance of omega-3 fats compared and omega-6 fats. Too many omega-6 fatty acids can reduce the body's ability to convert plant omega-3 into the important EPA and DHA omegas (see also pages 50–1 for more on the omega-3 and omega-6 balance). Both omega-3s and omega-6s are important though, and nuts, seeds and avocados give us omega-6. You can increase the omega-3 in your diet drastically by having ground flax seeds every day, which are more bioavailable than whole seeds. To be on the safe side, I would also suggest an algae-based EPA/DHA supplement if you are avoiding fish.

BREASTFEEDING

Your body will have a huge amount to deal with during childbirth and in the weeks afterwards. You will need to build up your body's nutrients like never before – to heal the wounds of childbirth or a Caesarean, to have the energy to care for your baby (and any other children/responsibilities you have) and to provide a food source for your new baby. Your hormonal changes will affect your mood, as will the inevitable sleep deprivation – and some women have pain while beginning to breastfeed too. Nutrition is one of the keys to boosting mood and resilience for you, and if you decide to breastfeed, your food will also help boost your baby's immune system and gut microbiome. An important part of your breastfeeding journey is immediately after birth when your milk starts to come in. Colostrum is thick and golden yellow in colour. It is dense in antibodies, setting up your baby's immune system.

When you are breastfeeding, you might notice your appetite increase. It's easy to be tempted to eat convenience and junk foods to satisfy your new appetite. But a great tip is to start off every day with a green smoothie using kale or spinach and fruits you enjoy, along with nut butter or avocado to make sure you give yourself a nutrient and water boost.

Drink lots of water to help avoid dehydration and boost your milk supply and this will also keep your bowels moving. In the early days, prioritise feeding your baby and getting lots of rest – there'll always be tidying up to do and exercise can wait for a while.

The decision to breastfeed is a personal one. And it really isn't all that easy for everyone – it is something that is supposed to be so natural and yet can sometimes be fraught with difficulty. Do not give yourself a hard time if it becomes an issue affecting your mental health – the baby needs a present and happy mum more than anything else. If you can do it – great. Breastmilk is amazing. You make the milk especially for your child, and its antibody content and nutrient density changes based on what your baby needs, each and every time they feed. Making sure they completely drain one side before starting feeding on the other is important as it may reduce the risk of mastitis.

Special receptors at the areola (around the nipple) send signals to let your body know exactly what antibodies your baby needs, you make them and pass them through your milk until such time as they can make their own. When your baby starts to 'cluster feed', which can often happen at around growth spurts, don't worry that you are not producing enough milk for them because your baby is doing this to stimulate further production. Unfortunately, most milk production occurs in the early hours of the morning, which can impact your sleep but is biologically normal.

Breastfeeding your baby until they are around six months old will mean they are less likely to get diarrhoea, vomiting and respiratory infections. But the benefits of breastfeeding last for far longer than six months, and the WHO suggests breastfeeding for as long as you can, to the age of two and beyond.

Why else is breastfeeding so uniquely helpful? Milk contains HMOs (human milk oligosaccharides) that provide nutrition not just for the baby, but to feed their microbes too. Unbelievably, these substances are present to nourish the billions of beneficial bugs that need to grow in your baby's gut for optimal health. There are 100 or more different HMOs needed to help your baby thrive.

For mothers, breastfeeding decreases the risk of breast cancer and it may also offer some protection against ovarian cancer. Breastmilk can continue to be given alongside an increasingly varied diet once your baby is introduced to solid foods. Babies up to one year of age who are being breastfed are advised to be given daily vitamin drops containing 8.5 to 10 micrograms (mcg) of vitamin D.

WHAT ABOUT FORMULA?

If you can't breastfeed and need to use formula that is OK. A fed baby and a healthy, happy mum is most important. What if you don't want to use cow's milk formula? A systematic review and meta-analysis from 2014 of the safety of soy-milk formulas found that 'the patterns of growth, bone health, and metabolic, reproductive endocrine, immune and neurological functions are similar to those fed human milk or cow's milk formula'.

Soy milk formulas have been used for decades and are especially useful for top-up feeds if mum is breastfeeding alongside formula. If you do decide to use a soy-based formula as the only milk your baby has before they are six months old, it is worth discussing it with a dietician. Because it will be their only nutrition, it is important to take your and your baby's medical history into account. There are some babies for whom soy milk will not be suitable. One thing that is important to know, is that any home-made baby formula is never a safe option. This should only be considered as a drink for babies over the age of one.

PHYTO-RICH KIDS

Almost one in five children are overweight or obese when they begin school, and one in three by the time they leave primary school. Obesity rates are highest in the most deprived 10 per cent of the population. We know that obesity is linked to an increased risk of heart disease, cancer and all causes of mortality. A well-planned WFPB approach can reduce the risk of developing heart disease, diabetes and cancer. But the most immediate advantage for kids is that WFPB diets are also likely to be associated with reduced risk of asthma, allergies and recurrent infections in childhood – so not only are you improving their health for today but also giving them a fantastic chance to reduce their health risks in the future.

ASTHMA

Asthma prevalence in kids has been rising steadily since the 1980s. Asthma now affects 5–10 per cent of the population or an estimated 23.4 million people, including 7 million children. This may in part be fuelled by increasing obesity, as well as increases in air pollution. But components of diet may also have something to do with this rise. And plants may help to provide a solution. I have had patients who have noticed that their children's asthma has improved on a WFPB diet, and who have even been able to cut down on or stop using their inhalers. This must always be done under medical supervision.

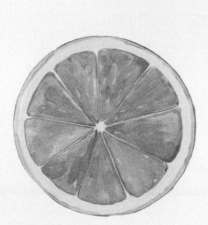
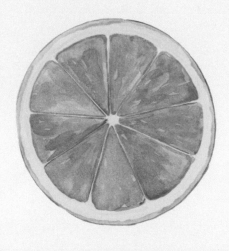

There are a few studies that can help us to see this is not just coincidence. One study looked at the immediate effects of milk on the lungs of asthma patients by serving them either a glass of whole milk, skimmed milk or water before assessing lung function. They looked at peak flow – a simple measurement to see how much air can be blown from the lungs – and did a test called DLCO (which stands for diffusion capacity of lungs for carbon monoxide). This is a test that determines how much oxygen travels from the alveoli of the lungs into the bloodstream. Although peak flow was not affected by cow's milk, the researchers found a progressive deterioration in the ability of the lungs to carry oxygen from whole milk to skimmed (via semi-skimmed).

Another study looked at dairy and eggs. They took 22 children with asthma and for two months half the children were given an egg- and dairy-free diet, and the other half stuck with their normal diets. The no egg and dairy group experienced a 22 per cent improvement in peak expiratory flow rate, while children following their normal diets experienced a slight reduction in peak flow. Meanwhile, a case-control study on 287 Peruvian children with asthma reported reduced likelihood of asthma with increased consumption of fruit, vegetables, legumes, cereals, pasta, rice and potatoes, and reduced meat intake.

In another study of 158 children with asthma, the more the kids stuck to a Mediterranean diet, the better their lung function. Plant predominant diets have also been shown to be helpful for other allergic disorders such as eczema. Hopefully, a plant-rich diet will also give your kids a great foundation for their adult lives too.

FUSSY KIDS

I get it, and I have been there – most parents feel so much anxiety around making sure their children have eaten enough. This is especially relevant for kids on the autistic spectrum, for whom routine, texture and familiarity are so important.

Be kind to yourself and remember it can take many attempts for a child to like a new taste. Do not let it become a battle of wills or you will find that your child wins – or that you win at the expense of your relationship with them.

Keep it simple – you choose what meals to serve, and they choose how much they eat. A relaxed dinnertime is definitely easier said than done, but consistently giving healthy meals to the whole family and trying to avoid stress if your son or daughter turns it away is crucial. Get them involved with food prep if you have time, or perhaps offer them the choice of two meals for which you have the ingredients, so they feel involved in the plan.

Kids are remarkably efficient at knowing when they are full, so don't worry too much if they don't eat what you have given them every single meal. I often used to give much bigger portions than my kids needed and would worry when they didn't eat it all. Look at the size of your child's hand to help guide you on the amount of food to give them; wholegrains should be equal to about a fist, and total fruit or veggie portions should be a couple of palms' worth (not counting fingers). This might be less than you'd normally put on a plate. But a smaller plate is a much less daunting prospect at dinnertime for them, as well as being a more realistic approximation of their energy and nutrition needs for your peace of mind.

So how do you know your children are getting enough nutrients? It is important to make sure – especially if your child is used to the same foods every day – that they get the right amount of nutrients from foods, fortified foods and supplements. Growing children need lots of energy (calories), healthy fats and nutrients, and so a wide variety of vegetables, fruit, wholegrains, legumes, nuts and seeds will be important for meeting their nutritional needs. Examples of foods kids love include porridge oats with seeds and berries, hummus and fruit snacks, wholegrain toast and beans, a smoothie, tofu scramble or almond butter with apple dippers. More examples can be found in the recipe section (see pages 190–265).

PLANT-BASED SENIORS

We are never too old to start taking care of our health. In fact, what is the point of living to an old age if we can't continue to enjoy life and do the things we really love? So how can we optimise health as we get older to ensure we can stay active and happy? All the benefits of a WFPB diet are particularly useful as we age, because this is the time when health issues that we could ignore in our youth become more insistent and start to encroach upon our quality of life.

Chronic airway diseases, arthritis and debility can creep up on us. So many of my patients joke with me and say, 'Don't get old, doctor . . .' But with some basic tips combining quality diet with exercise, enough sleep and minimising stress, you can ensure that you live better for longer. Eating a WFPB diet can also slow down ageing on a cellular level by increasing telomerase, an enzyme that repairs the telomeres at the end of human DNA strands.

So, what do we need to know? As we age, our nutritional requirements change. Our need for macronutrients increases but we need fewer calories and our metabolism naturally slows. As we eat less, it is important to ensure all food is nutrient dense, so every bite counts. Protein-rich foods will be more important over the age of 65, to help reduce the muscle wasting that tends to occur in these later years.

It is important to maintain optimal levels of vitamin D and calcium to reduce the risk of fractures and osteoporosis. But it's not just about bone health – muscle cells have special receptors for vitamin D in their nucleus, which promote muscle growth and can also improve balance.

This is so important as we age because, on average, we lose 1 per cent of our muscle mass every year after the age of 40, and 30 per cent every decade after the age of 50. So adequate vitamin D will be important for muscle function too. What will good bone and muscle strength mean? A reduced risk of falls.

Falls are a leading cause of death in older people, as fractures lead to frailty, immobility and increased risk of blood clots and infections. Vitamin D deficiency is a recognised predictor of falls in older people, with associations between low vitamin D and muscle weakness, impaired balance and faster loss of muscle mass. This means having enough vitamin D can not only keep bones healthy and reduce the impact of a fall, but also reduce the risk of a fall occurring in the first place. I would advise you to find out your vitamin D levels, and if they have been low and are now optimised, a simple 1,000IU–2,000IU supplement daily to maintain your levels should be adequate.

Staying active into your dotage is one of the very best ways to help reduce the effects of ageing – it will improve your bone and muscle mass as well as your flexibility, brain function, balance and mood. Resistance exercise is also crucial, and so easily overlooked. It is not just for gym bunnies and using your own body weight if you don't have weights is a great way to avoid muscle wasting as you get older.

Vitamin B12 deficiency is common over the age of 50, whatever your diet habits. A common condition called atrophic gastritis can occur, which can reduce the amount of vitamin B12 you absorb. Medications that are commonly taken as we get older, including certain diabetes medications such as metformin, and stomach-acid-suppressing drugs, can also reduce how much B12 we absorb. Anyone on a plant-based diet will benefit from supplementing B12. In North America, the Institute of Medicine recommends that everyone aged 50 years and older should get their B12 from fortified foods or supplements, whatever they eat, as after this age we are not as able to cleave the B12 off of the protein it is bound to in animal products.

Other supplements that may be useful depending on your general health could be omega-3s and perhaps a general multivitamin including iodine and selenium too.

When transitioning to a WFPB diet, you can talk to your doctor if you notice that any foods or supplements you try are interacting with any medications you are taking. If you take medications for blood pressure or diabetes – especially insulin – they can monitor you closely and make the necessary adjustments.

FRAILTY AND FOOD

Many chronic conditions and medications may interfere with your appetite, digestion, nutrient absorption, hydration and swallowing. Other factors like fatigue, depression and loneliness may also make diet choices less of a priority. Diet is not a cure-all but eating this way should hopefully prevent some of these issues from arising if healthy habits are adopted before frailty occurs. This gives you a proactive choice and allows you to become the architect of your own health. When you are at a stage where you are struggling to get the appetite to eat well, or are at risk of swallowing problems or dehydration, this is not the best time to make changes – seek out help from a dietician, or ask your family to help you get a referral to a dietician, as you will benefit from bespoke nutritional advice from a healthcare professional.

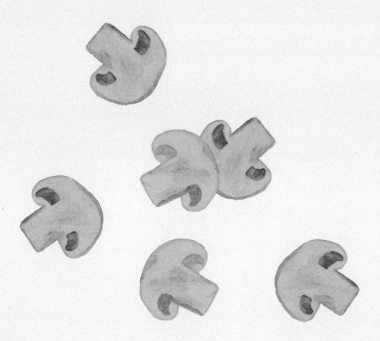

SUPPLEMENTS

I always prefer that we get as many of our nutrients from food as possible. Getting vitamin C, lycopene or iron in the form a pill is just not as good as eating the carrot, sun-dried tomato or broccoli. There is so much synergy from these foods, and phytonutrients present we have not even named yet. Add to this the fact that some supplements can be harmful in excess (such as vitamin A), and others give you expensive urine as you will process and pee out any excess.

However, it can sometimes be difficult to optimise nutrient intake through diet alone, especially if we have busy lives or financial restrictions. Some have said plant based eating is not natural because a vitamin B12 supplement is recommended. But anyone who eats shop-bought bread is receiving fortification of calcium, iron, niacin and thiamine. Anyone drinking cow's milk is receiving fortified iodine. Without realising it, we are technically eating supplements in our food all the time. As well as this, around half of us in the UK say we regularly take food supplements or vitamins – regardless of dietary preference. The truth is, all of us have key nutrients we should be mindful of, whatever we choose to eat. For example, people over the age of fifty are more prone to vitamin B12 deficiencies, as are those with coeliac disease or who drink heavily. Pregnant women are advised to take folate and are much more likely to be iron deficient, as are women with heavy periods. We all have key nutrients to consider. Fortunately, plant-based eaters are more likely to be abundant in beneficial nutrients such as fibre, antioxidants, magnesium, potassium and folate. However, just like omnivores, there are also key nutrients that people who eat a plant-based diet need to ensure they are getting.

VITAMIN B12

If you decide to eat a fully WFPB diet, that's wonderful. In this case, B12 supplementation will be essential. Luckily many foods are fortified with B12 now too. Where is vitamin B12 from? Vitamin B12 is made from soil microbes. Vitamin B12 doesn't originate in meat, but it is found cow, pig and chicken meat because they have eaten soil or drunk water containing these micro-organisms, or eaten corn feed with B12 supplements added to it.

Even people who eat a lot of meat and eggs will potentially be B12 deficient after the age of 50 as their stomach can have problems absorbing it (see page 179). Also, other medical factors such as taking certain medications, malabsorption issues and autoimmune disorders can reduce absorption of vitamin B12. So, it's a good idea to check your levels and supplement, especially for diabetics. Don't take the risk of avoiding supplementation or adequate amounts of fortified foods – it's far better to be safe than sorry.

There are many different types of vitamin B (thiamin, riboflavin, niacin, B6, biotin and folate) which are abundant in a WFPB diet. Although many foods are fortified with B12 now (plant milks, Marmite, nutritional yeast), for ease of ensuring you have enough, B12 supplementation makes sense.

UK guidelines state that adults only need about 1.5mcg vitamin B12 a day. However, I'd recommend taking at least 10mcg daily or 2,000mcg a week. If you take a weekly supplement, the dose is higher because the body absorbs less. In North America, the RDA is 2.4mcg, but some experts now believe adults can benefit from 4–7mcg of vitamin D for optimal B12 status, and a supplement as high as 500–1,000mcg per day if you are over the age of 65. These recommendations are safe and will ensure you have enough not only to prevent deficiency, but to also reliably break down an amino acid called homocysteine, which in excess causes oxidative stress and is implicated in a higher risk of heart attacks and strokes. Your body absorbs vitamin B12 more efficiently in frequent small amounts, so the less often you have it, the more you need.

VITAMIN D

The only way to reliably get enough vitamin D other than through sun exposure is with a supplement. This is because it is not that readily available from food. As mentioned, a WFPB approach avoids fish, eggs and cod liver oil, and the only plant sources are mushrooms that have been sunbathing – yes, brown mushrooms – and fortified foods, such as plant milks and cereals. But remember only around 10 per cent of our vitamin D needs can be absorbed through diet. Even if you eat a healthy diet, you still may become vitamin D deficient.

The Scientific Advisory Committee for Nutrition (SACN) recommends vitamin D supplementation as follows:

- Breastfed babies up to one year old should have a daily supplement containing 8.5 to 10 micrograms of vitamin D.

- Formula-fed babies should not get a supplement until they are having less than 500ml infant formula a day (infant formula is fortified with vitamin D).

- Children aged one to four should get a daily supplement containing 10 micrograms of vitamin D.

- For adults and children over four, it is recommended that they consider a daily supplement containing 10 micrograms during autumn and winter.

However, there are some of us who may need more, such as the elderly, people who work in office environments, people who cover up in the sun and people with dark skin, who may not absorb enough vitamin D. These people should consider a vitamin D supplement all year round. If in doubt, always talk to your doctor. Getting your quota of vitamin D could help to improve your bone, immune and mental health, and is such an easy win when it comes to lifestyle change. I'd recommend at least 1,000iu a day in those who have normal levels, and 2,000iu a day if you have a tendency to run low. If you are already deficient you could need higher doses. UK advice is for 10mcg (400iu) for everyone in winter and all year round for at risk groups, without the need to check levels.

OTHER SUPPLEMENTS

- **Algae oil**
  EPA/DHA supplements can be useful. These are the purest form of long-chain omega-3 fatty acids on the planet. Made from algae, where fish get it from too, it means you can consider supplementing without taking cod liver oil and avoiding the heavy metals and toxins in fish.

- **Flax seeds**
  These are a superfood and definitely worth having every day. One to two tablespoons of milled flax every day will help keep your blood vessels supple and could also drop your blood pressure and boost heart health. Mix into your

morning porridge, sprinkle in a salad or main meal, add it to your smoothie or even bake with it (one tablespoon in three tablespoons of water can replace one egg in baking).

Iodine

Plant-based sources include seaweed and fortified foods. Seaweed has highly variable and unreliable amounts (dulce and nori sheets used in sushi are better choices than kelp), so it's not recommended to have every day. Many plant milks are now supplemented with iodine like cow's milk, but you must check the label. You might wish to consider a non-seaweed supplement.

Selenium

The amount of selenium in a plant varies depending on how much is in the soil it is grown in. Brazil nuts are famous for their high levels, and one or two nuts a day are likely to be enough.

Zinc

Zinc can be obtained by eating a balanced diet of pulses (especially baked beans), grains (oats), vegetables, nuts and seeds. Nutritional yeast flakes are a great source of zinc and are often a source of vitamin B12 too. Top tip – onion and garlic can both increase your absorption of zinc from foods so be sure to cook with them to maximise your zinc and iron.

Always ensure you buy your supplements from reputable retailers and sources.

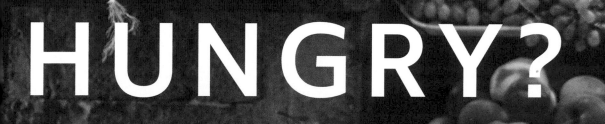

HUNGRY?

A NEW WAY TO EAT

Sometimes thinking about making a wholescale change to your lifestyle can feel overwhelming. Many of us have tried fad diets in the past or promised ourselves we were going to succeed with a massive health kick, only to feel crushingly disappointed when we fail. You are doing nothing wrong. You are not weak willed.

This is no 7-day challenge. There is no 360-degree programme. And this is definitely not a fad. Instead, all I ask is that you promise yourself to start by just doing one thing and feel really good about it.

Professor BJ Fogg at Stanford discusses behaviour change science in terms of a garden analogy, which of course I love! He encourages people to think of habits as like seeds that must be planted to make a garden. Sometimes it is just the wrong spot in the garden, or the wrong time of year for a habit seed to turn into a habit plant. Where does this new habit fit best in your garden? How can it take root for you?

The fact you are reading this book suggests you are open to starting a new habit. This open-mindedness will help you hardwire the habit and builds what is known as 'success momentum'. The more we feel good about ourselves, the more we want to do to feel even better. Although many of you will want to jump in and try 100 per cent WFPB eating, if at some point you don't eat from the WFPB shopping list, don't beat yourself up. Celebrate what you've done to nurture your habit garden, and don't get bogged down with being perfect.

Let's stop with the self-criticism. Notice when you are hard on yourself and instead think about what a good friend would say. I want this book to feel like that for you.

WHAT IS IMPORTANT TO YOU?

Ask yourself these three questions:

What things are important to you that you must include in your life?

These could be single words or concepts.

Examples are – joy, fun, health, family. These are just examples. Write down all the ones you can think of that are important to you.

What are your top three?

What do you currently have or do in your life that aligns with your key values?

So, if health is in your top three and you already walk the dog each day that can be on your list. If family comes first, notice all the ways in which you prioritise them in your day to day as of this moment. Your list will be unique to you, because your top three values are unique to you. Write down as many things you do now – or have done in the past – that align with your top three values.

When you can't think of any more you can come back to it later and add any that you remember. Look at the list. Here comes the fun part – I want you to allow yourself to feel a sense of celebration, and a sense of joy. There is probably a lot on the list that you had not noticed. Feel proud of it all.

How would a WFPB diet fit with your key values?

Think here about any simple changes that will bring you more of the health, happiness or peace of mind that you need. This is a good way of noticing what comes to mind for you.

When you wake up each morning, you can repeat your three values out loud, or under your breath. This will take less than five seconds. But it will remind you why you are doing what you do. Whatever your day holds, it is a simple thing to keep you feeling good about yourself and what you believe. The rest will flow from there.

When you notice yourself doing something that honours one of your three things, take the time to say well done. Whether it is in your head, or out loud, whatever works for you. Just acknowledge that you had a choice, and you chose to do something to bring you better health and happiness. That deserves to be celebrated. Daily wins can turn into weekly habits, which turn into a lifetime of changes you can feel truly proud of.

MY PATIENTS' TOP TIPS

I am going to share some of the simple switches my patients have told me helped them to feel better.

Plan your meals before you start

One patient even did his own spreadsheet that he filled in each day. He was a computer engineer, and structure and routine were important values to him! If you want to plan your meals, you can use the meal planner on page 298. Make sure you have all the staples you need to succeed in the cupboard before you start.

Keep things easy

If you know you will be starving after arriving home from work, for example, choose an easy option. One of my patients decided to take a packet of marinated tofu from the shop and mix with sweetcorn and plant-based mayonnaise she had made the day before so she had a few days of sandwich fillings done in advance.

Don't demand perfection

Do what is sustainable for your lifestyle. If you don't feel like cooking, choose a vegetable and hummus sandwich, or another healthy, no-cook choice. Beans and wholemeal toast will do just fine if you are tired.

Enlist support

Tell your family and friends that you are making some changes. Don't be afraid to seek support from others. One of my diabetic patients started to do really well with his blood sugar control when his wife learned to cook some plant-based recipes and they did it together. If you have resistant family or friends, you can find a support network online – meet-ups, local support groups, Facebook groups and more.

Start with milk

One of my asthmatic patients swapped out cow's milk for a plant milk as a first step. She said it was fun to try different ones and discover a type that she liked.

One meal a day

Actress Suzie Cameron and her film director husband James Cameron swear by the 'OMD' technique. This means making one meal each day 100 per cent plant based and committing to that. One of my patients found this really helpful and decided her OMD would be breakfast. For her, that meant a routine of wholegrain cereal and granola with plant milk, berries and seeds, and on the weekend, avocado on toast and plant-based pancakes.

Just one more

My friend, GP and author Dr Rupy Aujla, talks about the concept of adding 'just one more' vegetable to each meal to make it easier to get healthy. If you are having a curry, chuck in some spinach to wilt into it. If you are having a sandwich, add in some cucumber and a dollop of hummus on the side. One of my patients uses a rainbow chart to help remind her and her children to add in one more vegetable each day, which was a great tip from my lovely friend and author Dr Rangan Chatterjee.

Soy solution

This tip came from one of my menopausal patients who realised that soy products helped with her flushing. She promised herself she would have one soy product a day, every day. For her, this meant edamame beans, soy milk, tofu or tempeh. This worked well for her.

Simple swaps

My favourite tip came from one of my patients who was a self-confessed vegetable-phobe. He loved chilli con carne and beefburgers and so he decided he would start with a simple swap. He got a veggie mince and a fake meat burger that tasted as good as the real thing as his first step. Then after a few weeks he decided to make a three-bean chilli instead and try a peanut butter and bean burger. After a few more weeks, he realised his cravings for beefburgers had gone. He tried to eat one, bit into it . . . and it felt like a huge disappointment. It just didn't taste the same. It was at that moment he felt a sudden sense of pride. He told me, 'I knew then that I was a veggie lover!' I would encourage an all-in approach, but if this feels like too big a leap, a few gentler steps can help you get there.

YOUR PLANT-POWERED KITCHEN

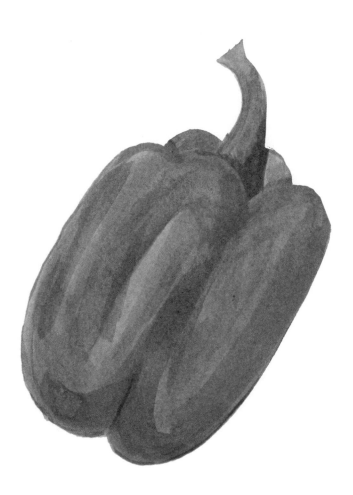

ESSENTIAL INGREDIENTS

Are you confused about what you need in your cupboards to get started on your plant power journey? Do you want to be able to make these recipes without rushing to the shops to buy just one or two key ingredients? Then simply use this store cupboard ingredients list to guide you. This list gives you the basics for a zero-hassle meal every time.

DRY INGREDIENTS AND TINS

Oats
Pearled barley
Wholemeal pasta
Wholewheat noodles
Wholemeal bread
Tortillas
Chopped tomatoes
Passata
Black beans
Chickpeas
Cannellini beans
Butter beans
Tinned artichoke hearts
Tinned jackfruit
Coconut milk
Coconut cream
Brown lentils
Cooked chestnuts
Red wine (optional)

HERBS AND SPICES

Dried oregano
Dried mint
Dried tarragon
Dried parsley
Bay leaves
Garlic powder
Mustard powder
Smoked paprika
Chinese 5 spice
Cardamon pods
Cinnamon sticks
Ground cinnamon
Ground ginger
Ground turmeric
Ground cumin
Ground coriander
Cumin seeds
Coriander seeds
Mustard seeds
Garam masala or spices of your choice
Curry powder
Smoked chilli powder (optional)

SAUCES AND CONDIMENTS

BBQ or chipotle sauce
Tamari or light soy sauce
Rice wine vinegar
Vegan balsamic vinegar
Cider vinegar
Mustard
Tahini
Miso paste
Lemon juice
Tomato purée
Liquid smoke
Olive oil (optional)
Molasses
Vegetable stock
Mushroom stock
Nutritional yeast
Marmite
Black olives
Capers
Gherkins
Apricot jam
Pineapple juice

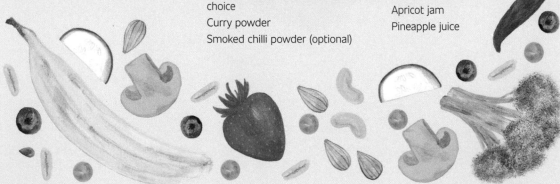

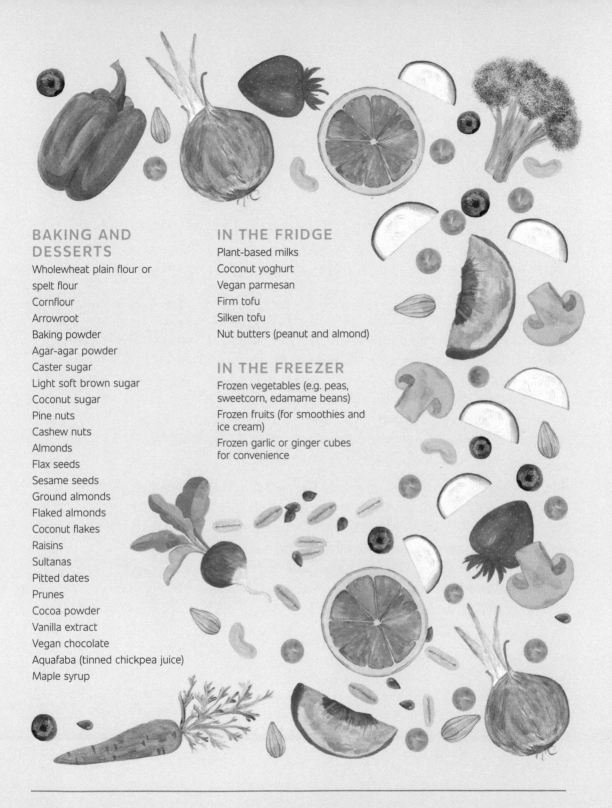

BAKING AND DESSERTS

Wholewheat plain flour or spelt flour
Cornflour
Arrowroot
Baking powder
Agar-agar powder
Caster sugar
Light soft brown sugar
Coconut sugar
Pine nuts
Cashew nuts
Almonds
Flax seeds
Sesame seeds
Ground almonds
Flaked almonds
Coconut flakes
Raisins
Sultanas
Pitted dates
Prunes
Cocoa powder
Vanilla extract
Vegan chocolate
Aquafaba (tinned chickpea juice)
Maple syrup

IN THE FRIDGE

Plant-based milks
Coconut yoghurt
Vegan parmesan
Firm tofu
Silken tofu
Nut butters (peanut and almond)

IN THE FREEZER

Frozen vegetables (e.g. peas, sweetcorn, edamame beans)
Frozen fruits (for smoothies and ice cream)
Frozen garlic or ginger cubes for convenience

BREAKFAST

It's really important to get the day started with a healthy and nutritious breakfast. Whether you are feeding your family or yourself, a good breakfast will kick-start your body and fuel you through the day. In this section, I have included recipes that can be adapted with a variety of options to suit your tastes and the seasons.

I love cooking with oats as an everyday staple. Whole oats are high in beta-glucans which is great for reducing cholesterol, improving blood sugars and balancing your immune system. Oats also contain phenolic acids which offer antioxidant and anti-inflammatory protection. Avenanthramides are antioxidants in oats that help reduce skin irritation too! Packed with fibre, vitamins and minerals (such as thiamine, magnesium, zinc and selenium), you can boost the protein content of your oats by adding a swirl of almond butter to your bowl.

The best oats? The least processed. The 'wholegrain hierarchy' for oats goes something like this: oat groats, oat bran, steel cut, rolled oats and instant oats. Though be warned, oat groats will need soaking overnight and will remain a bit chewy. All oats are healthy, but steel cut or rolled are probably the healthiest choices without having to soak them in advance.

I am also a massive fan of pancakes as a treat at the weekends or on special days. My family love them and they can be made with a whole host of different WFPB toppings, so they are full of nutrients and taste amazing.

PANCAKES

Basic recipe will make
20–24 pancakes, can
easily be halved, enough
for 4–6 portions

300g plain flour
(preferably wholemeal or
spelt or a combination)

1 tbsp baking powder

½ tsp bicarbonate of soda

500ml plant-based milk
(soy or oat are best)

2 tbsp lemon juice or cider
apple vinegar

1 tbsp date or maple syrup
(optional)

1 tsp vanilla extract

Salt

What could be nicer on a weekend morning than whipping up a batch of pancakes? These ones are light and fluffy and perfect as part of a lazy breakfast or brunch.

Whisk the flour with the baking powder, bicarbonate of soda and a pinch of salt. Mix the milk and lemon juice or cider apple vinegar together and leave to stand until the milk thickens. Stir in the syrup, if using, and the vanilla extract.

Pour the wet ingredients into the dry, and mix, but don't over-mix as this will make the pancakes tough – a few lumps are fine.

Heat a non-stick or well-seasoned cast-iron frying pan until fairly hot. Ladle rounds of the batter into the pan – around 4 at a time. Leave them to cook until large bubbles appear on the top and they look as though they are setting round the edges. Flip the pancakes carefully (a metal spatula works best, though if you're using a non-stick pan, be careful not to scratch it), and cook the other sides until lightly brown. Repeat with the remaining batter in 5–6 batches.

TURN OVER FOR SEASONAL VARIATIONS

BANANA PANCAKES

Add 2 mashed bananas to the batter, serve with syrup and more sliced bananas or berries.

SPICED RAISIN

Add 1 tsp mixed spice and ½ tsp ground cinnamon to the dry ingredients. Soak 100g raisins or sultanas in boiled water or hot tea for 5 minutes and drain. Sprinkle a few on top of the pancakes when you have ladled them out. Serve with sweetened vegan cream cheese and syrup.

TOASTED COCONUT

Toast 50g desiccated coconut in a dry frying pan until lightly coloured, then cool and add to the dry ingredients. Serve with coconut yoghurt (optional), slices of mango or papaya and a squeeze of lime juice.

OAT AND APPLE

Toast 50g oats in a dry frying pan until lightly coloured and aromatic. Proceed as in the main recipe on page 195. Take 2 eating apples and slice into wedges. Arrange over a dry frying pan and sprinkle with ground cinnamon or mixed spice. Add a tablespoon or two of water and heat gently until browned on one side, then flip and cook the other side. Serve with the pancakes and a drizzle of maple syrup, if you like.

TAHINI/NUT BUTTER AND CHOCOLATE

Add 2 tbsp of well-mixed tahini or nut butter to the wet ingredients and whisk thoroughly. Proceed as in the main recipe on page 195. For the sauce: heat 200ml plant-based milk in a saucepan. Whisk in 1 tbsp maple syrup, 2 tbsp cocoa, 2 tbsp tahini or nut butter and 4 squares of dark chocolate until you have a smooth, pourable sauce.

A SAVOURY VERSION

Omit the vanilla extract. Blitz 50g spinach or kale with the milk and proceed as in the main recipe on page 195. Serve with Tofu Bacon Slices (see page 205) and a little maple syrup.

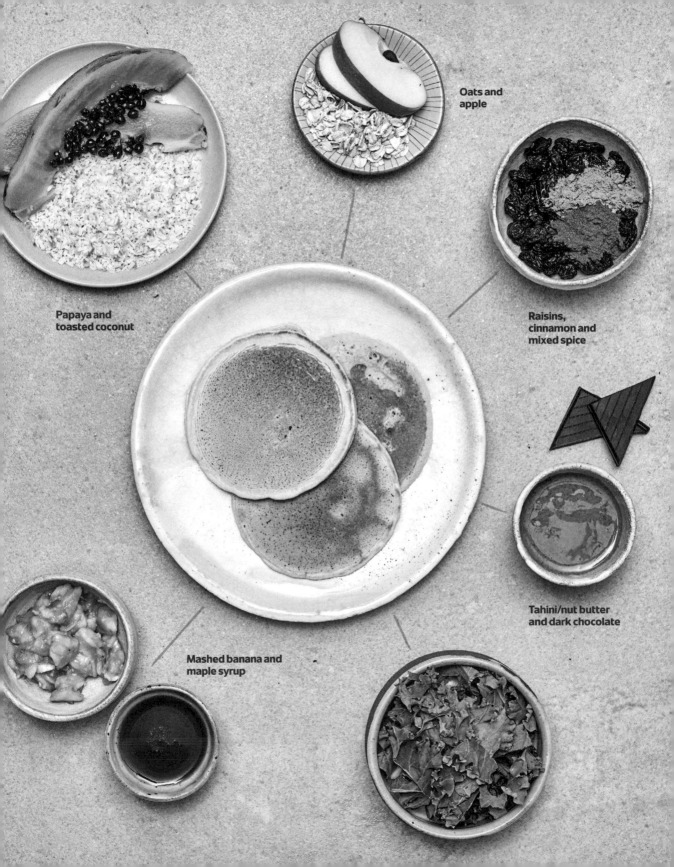

Oats and apple

Papaya and toasted coconut

Raisins, cinnamon and mixed spice

Tahini/nut butter and dark chocolate

Mashed banana and maple syrup

PORRIDGE

Makes 1 portion

40g porridge oats

360ml plant-based milk
(preferably oat) or water
if you want to do it the
Scottish way

Salt

Gone are the days when porridge was stodgy or boring – oats done right are the breakfast of champions!

Put the oats and the milk or water into a saucepan and set over a low to medium heat. Let the liquid gradually come up to just under the boil, stirring regularly, then continue to cook, stirring constantly until the oats have swelled and thickened the liquid – the consistency should be thick but pourable.

CHOCOLATE PORRIDGE

Add either 1 tbsp cocoa to the saucepan with the oats and cook as above, or serve the porridge with 1 square of vegan dark chocolate to be stirred in. Add 1 tbsp maple or date syrup, if you like.

TOASTED ALMONDS OR LARGE SEEDS

Toast 1 tbsp almonds, walnuts, coconut flakes or pumpkin seeds in a dry frying pan, stirring until they smell very nutty and have lightly browned. Scatter over or mix into the finished porridge. Serve with a drizzle of maple or date syrup.

GRAINS

Add 1 tsp each of as many different seeds as you like – quinoa (well rinsed), flax seeds, chia seeds, sesame seeds, poppy seeds – to the saucepan with the oats. Toast for several minutes until they give off a nutty aroma then add the milk. Continue as above.

FROZEN FRUITS

Frozen berries, either singly or in mixes (e.g. fruits of the forest), can be defrosted and stirred into porridge. Add around 2 tbsp defrosted fruit per serving. Add a little cinnamon for extra sweetness. Or simply add a couple of tablespoons of fruit compote.

AUTUMN FRUITS

Grate a chunk of pumpkin, an apple or pear and add to the porridge at the beginning of the cooking time with a pinch of cinnamon and ground ginger. Scatter over 1 tbsp of dried fruit (dates, raisins, prunes) to serve. Some powdered lucuma is really good with this too – add around 1 tbsp per serving.

OVERNIGHT OATS

Soaking your oats overnight in your chosen plant milk helps the starches to break down and may help you use their nutrients more effectively as well as giving a creamier taste. Soaking chia seeds overnight in the oats will also thicken the oats and add some omega-3s to your morning meal! Best of all, this will last several days in the fridge so you can tuck in whenever you want. Adding in a favourite teabag to soak, such as a chai blend, will add even more flavour. Try your favourite and see.

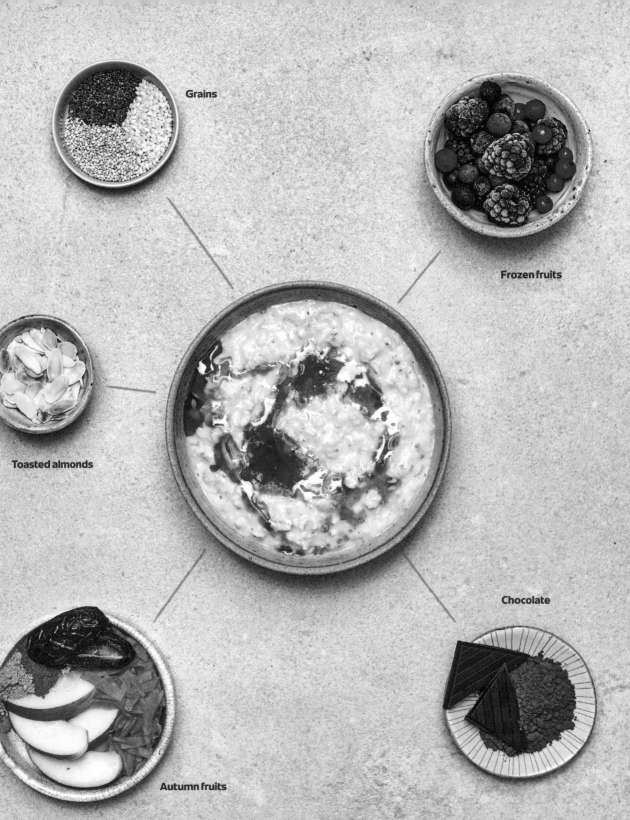

Grains

Frozen fruits

Toasted almonds

Chocolate

Autumn fruits

TOAST

Do you wonder what to put on your toast instead of butter or cheese? These delicious choices will make breakfast, lunch or tea more exciting and packed with WFPB goodness. Tomatoes and Marmite is my absolute favourite – you will never look back!

AVOCADO
Juice 1 lime into a bowl and add a pinch of salt. Mash in the avocado. Rub the wholemeal toast with half a garlic clove (optional), then spread on the avocado. Sprinkle with a little smoked chilli powder for a spicy kick.

TOMATOES
Spread the wholemeal toast with Marmite. Put 100g cherry tomatoes into a saucepan with a splash of water and simmer gently until they plump up. Squish onto the toast and top with a sprinkling of salt, pepper and dried oregano.

NUT BUTTER AND BANANA
Spread the wholemeal toast with any nut butter, then top with slices of banana.

VEGAN CREAMY SPREAD
Stir 1 tsp maple or date syrup, a few drops of vanilla extract and 1 tbsp soaked raisins or sultanas into vegan cream cheese. For extra crunch, add toasted nuts or seeds, or a handful of vegan granola.

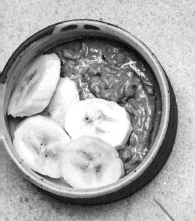

Nut butter and banana

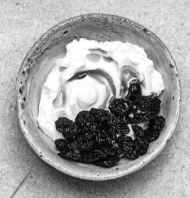

Raisins and vegan cream cheese

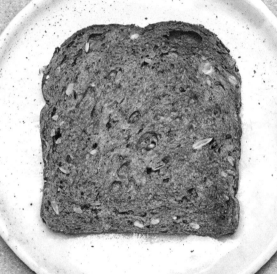

Tomatoes

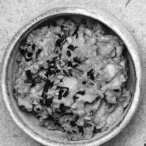

Avocado

Date syrup

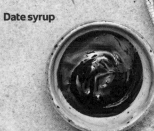

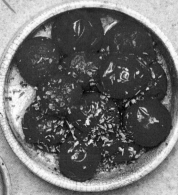

COOKED BREAKFAST

Makes 4 portions

Any combination of the following:

- Tofu Scramble
- Mushrooms and Tomatoes
- Bubble and Squeak
- Tofu Bacon Slices

Makes 4 portions

400g firm tofu (extra firm if you like a very firm scramble)

4 spring onions, finely sliced

Up to 100ml vegetable stock or water

2 tbsp nutritional yeast (optional)

¼ tsp ground turmeric

½ tsp garlic powder

2 tbsp finely chopped tarragon or parsley

200g baby leaf spinach or any cooked greens (optional)

Salt and pepper

A cooked breakfast can be the perfect way to start the day, so switch out your bacon and eggs for any combination of the following recipes. Here you can find all the WFPB inspiration you need to cook up a weekend feast.

If you want to include a vegan shop-bought sausage, look at the labels. For a healthier choice, pick products with more greens and ambers, avoiding any products with red labels and look for ones with the fewest number of ingredients.

TOFU SCRAMBLE

If the tofu has a lot of water, first prepare it by pressing it – simply place it between 2 plates and put a couple of tins on top – make sure you put a cloth around it to catch the water. Leave to stand for at least an hour and regularly strain off any liquid. Break up the tofu so it looks crumbled.

Put the tofu and spring onions into a dry frying pan and add a tablespoon of the stock. Fry for a few minutes, stirring constantly and adding a little more stock if the tofu is getting dry, until the spring onions have softened and the tofu is taking on a little colour.

Add the nutritional yeast (if using), turmeric and garlic powder, season with salt and pepper and pour in any remaining stock. Simmer, stirring regularly, until the liquid is absorbed and the tofu has taken on the colour of the turmeric – this should take about 4–5 minutes. Stir in the fresh herbs.

If adding spinach, wash thoroughly, then while still wet, wilt down in a separate pan. Drain thoroughly and stir through the tofu. Don't be tempted to add directly to the tofu as it will give out a lot of water and you will need to cook it until it has evaporated.

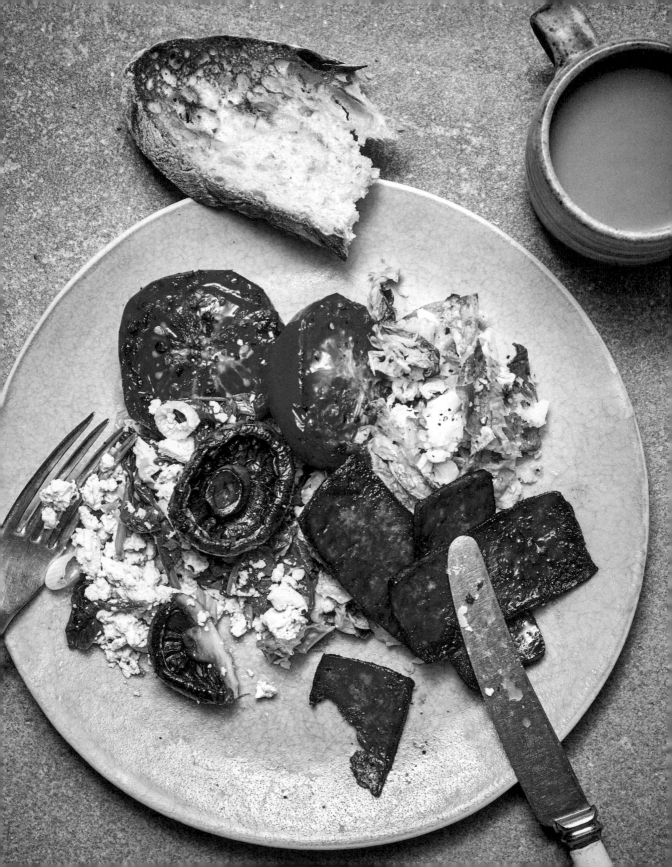

Makes 4 portions

4 medium tomatoes, halved horizontally

8 large white or chestnut mushrooms, halved

½ tsp dried oregano

Salt and pepper

MUSHROOMS AND TOMATOES

Put 2 tbsp water in a frying pan. When it is piping hot and starting to steam, add the tomatoes and mushrooms, cut side up, and season with salt, pepper and the dried oregano. Cook over a medium heat, adding more water as it evaporates off, until you can tell that the tomatoes are starting to soften and the mushrooms have taken on a little colour. Flip over and continue to cook, adding more water as necessary, until the tomatoes are cooked through and the cut sides have started to lightly caramelise, and the mushrooms have taken on a light golden brown colour.

Makes 4 portions

150g cabbage, shredded

300g cooked white potatoes, skin on, roughly chopped or crushed

Salt and pepper

BUBBLE AND SQUEAK

Preheat your oven to 180°C/350°F/gas mark 4. Wash the cabbage thoroughly then, without draining, put in a saucepan over a high heat. Cover and leave to wilt down. Drain thoroughly.

Mash the potatoes a little so that they're rough but not completely smooth. Combine with the cabbage and season with salt and pepper, then pile into an ovenproof dish. Bake in the preheated oven for around 20 minutes or until the top is crisp and lightly browned.

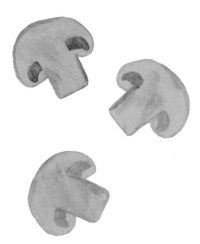

Makes 4 portions

100g smoked tofu, thinly sliced into strips

For the marinade

2 tbsp maple syrup

2 tbsp soy sauce

½ tsp garlic powder

¼ tsp paprika or chilli powder

A few drops of liquid smoke (optional – this can be bought in some supermarkets and health food shops too – it will change your life!)

Salt and pepper

TOFU BACON SLICES

I love tofu bacon and while you can buy strips of Quorn® or other substitute meat cut as bacon, I find the homemade version made from smoked tofu is amazing.

Mix all the marinade ingredients together and season with salt and pepper. Add the tofu slices, carefully submerging in the marinade, then leave to stand for 5 minutes.

Heat a non-stick frying pan and add the marinated tofu slices, frying them on both sides until they are crisp and brown. Pour any marinade over and keep turning the slices until they are glossy and well coated.

SMOOTHIES AND SMOOTHIE BOWLS

Makes 1 portion

1 large handful of spinach, kale or watercress (around 25–30g)

50g chunk of cucumber

1 apple, stem removed, roughly chopped

1 pear, stem removed, roughly chopped

1 kiwifruit, roughly chopped

10g flaked coconut, almonds, oats or seeds

A sprig of mint

6 ice cubes

A splash of water or plant-based milk to thin if necessary

To turn into a bowl

A handful of berries or grapes

1 tbsp flaked coconut or almonds

1 tbsp seeds

These smoothies and smoothie bowls are full of nutrients and flavour. This is enough to make one glass or bowl, but can easily be increased to make more. My kids prefer this as a drink and I've included easily obtainable fruit and vegetables. If you are making a smoothie, the fruit and veg will need to be unpeeled. (NB: with the kiwifruit, if you have a high-speed blender, you don't need to peel them. But if you want to be on the safe side, then peel the kiwi!)

Put all the ingredients for the smoothie into a blender and blitz until completely smooth. Check the consistency and add a little water or plant-based milk if you feel it needs thinning out – if you are making a smoothie bowl it is better to leave it thicker; for a drink, you may want to thin it down.

Pour into a glass or a bowl. For a smoothie bowl, top with fruit, almonds and seeds.

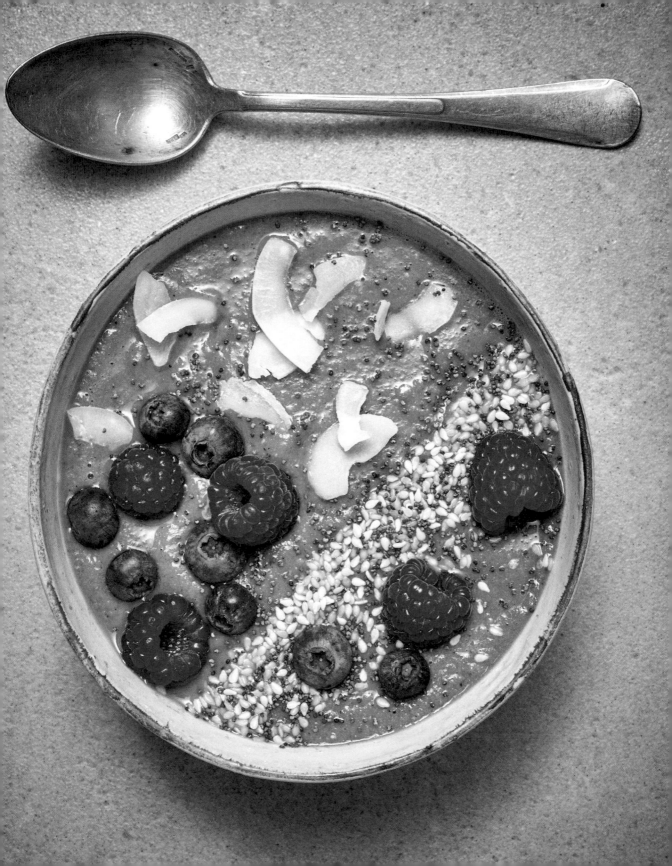

LUNCH

Are you stuck in a lunch rut and looking for inspiration?

Whether we are at work or at home, we tend to automatically reach for the same options. It can be really beneficial to plan a healthy and nutritious lunch and will also save you time and money. I've found that thinking about and packing my lunch the night before, while I am preparing or clearing up dinner, means that I can grab it on the way out the door. This section includes some of my lunchtime favourites and I hope to inspire you with a choice of sandwich fillings, soups and salads. I love to keep things simple but varied and always try to include a range of textures and tastes.

NO TUNA SANDWICH

Makes 4 generous sandwiches

For the chickpea mix

1 x 400g tin chickpeas

Zest and juice of 1 lemon

1 tbsp Dijon mustard

1 tbsp capers, finely chopped

1 tbsp gherkins or cornichons, finely chopped

1 tbsp olives, finely chopped

2 spring onions, finely chopped

1 stick celery, finely chopped

A few tarragon leaves, finely chopped (optional)

100g cooked sweetcorn

Salt and pepper

For the sandwich

8 slices wholemeal bread

½ cucumber, thinly sliced

A handful of rocket leaves

Vegan mayo (optional)

It can sometimes be hard to know what to put on your sarnie but this option is mouth-watering and packed full of nutrients! I love cornichons – mini gherkin cucumbers – they are absolutely delicious.

Put the chickpeas, lemon zest and juice and mustard into a food processor and pulse until the chickpeas have broken down and look creamy. You can also use a potato masher for this. Stir in all the remaining ingredients and season with salt and pepper. The mixture should be quite firm.

Spoon the chickpea mixture over 4 slices of bread and top with the cucumber and rocket leaves. Add vegan mayo if you like. Top with the remaining slices of bread and serve.

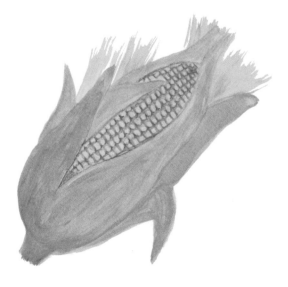

CLASSIC BLT

Makes 4 generous sandwiches

300g (preferably smoked) tofu, thinly sliced, marinated and cooked (see page 205)

2 avocados, mashed

Juice of ½ lime

8 slices wholemeal bread

2 ripe tomatoes, thinly sliced

Lettuce – Iceberg, Cos or Romaine

Salt and pepper

There is nothing like a juicy BLT sandwich and is here is my version with tofu instead of bacon (see page 205 for the tofu bacon recipe). I've also replaced the mayonnaise or butter with mashed avocado.

Fry the tofu slices and set aside. Mash the avocado with the lime juice and plenty of seasoning. Spread the avocado on all 8 slices of bread. Layer the tofu, tomato and lettuce onto 4 slices of the bread and top with the remaining slices. Cut in half and serve.

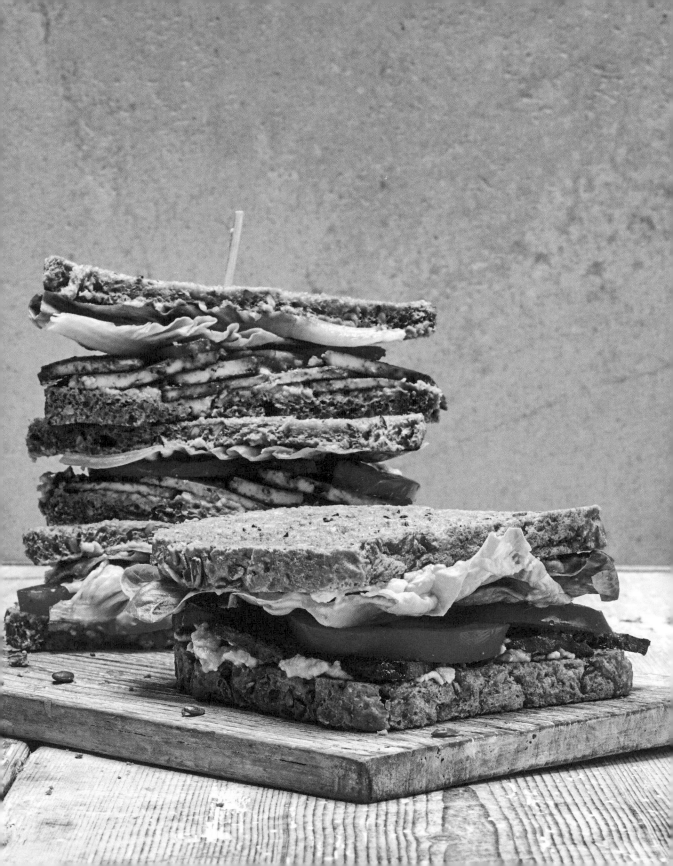

SANDWICH FILLINGS

Sandwiches are cheap, quick to make and great for eating on the go. Here are some suggestions to brighten up your lunchbox!

PEANUT BUTTER AND JAM

PB and J is a classic sandwich, but for a healthier twist grated apple or mashed banana are really tasty in place of the jam. You could even try crushing up some fresh berries if you want! Strawberries and raspberries work well, and you can add a sprinkle of sugar. Make sure you spread both sides of the bread with peanut butter and crush the fruit on a board so you can strain away excess juice – otherwise the bread will be soggy.

BEETROOT, WATERCRESS AND HORSERADISH

(Not the creamed sauce, make sure it's vegan.) Spread the horseradish sauce over the bread and follow with thinly sliced beetroot and watercress. This is also good with smoked tofu.

FALAFEL

Try these (oven baked) sliced in a sandwich or wholemeal pitta, with lettuce, cucumber, tomato and a roast red pepper tahini dressing – purée a roast red pepper with 2 tbsp tahini, the juice of ½ lemon and 1 garlic clove. Add chilli for a hotter dressing. This is also good drizzled over hummus in a sandwich.

RAINBOW SANDWICH

Include thinly sliced tomato, grated carrot, yellow pepper, sliced avocado or lettuce, thinly sliced radish or shredded red cabbage. With the avocado you don't need any other dressing.

CARROT HUMMUS WITH RAISINS OR SEEDS

Take a portion of hummus, blitz with a grated carrot and pinches of ground turmeric, cumin and cinnamon. Stir through a sprinkle of raisins or pomegranate seeds and pumpkin seeds. Serve in a sandwich with salad greens.

ROCKET, TOMATO AND VEGAN PARMESAN

Dress the rocket with a very little vegan balsamic vinegar, then layer with tomato and some shredded vegan cheese.

PEA PESTO

Make a pesto by blitzing 100g blanched peas with a little lemon juice, 1 tsp dried mint and 25g pine nuts. Use as a sandwich spread and add plenty of greens – lots of peppery cress would work with this.

CURRIED CAULIFLOWER

Blanch cauliflower for 1 minute. Toss in your favourite curry powder and chilli powder, a tbsp of oil if using, and roast for 15 minutes. Slice and serve in a sandwich with a raita made from cashew cream (for the recipe, see the coleslaw on page 230), ½ tsp nigella seeds, ½ grated and strained cucumber, a squeeze of lime juice and plenty of finely chopped fresh mint. Add a little hot sauce to the sandwich if you like it spicy.

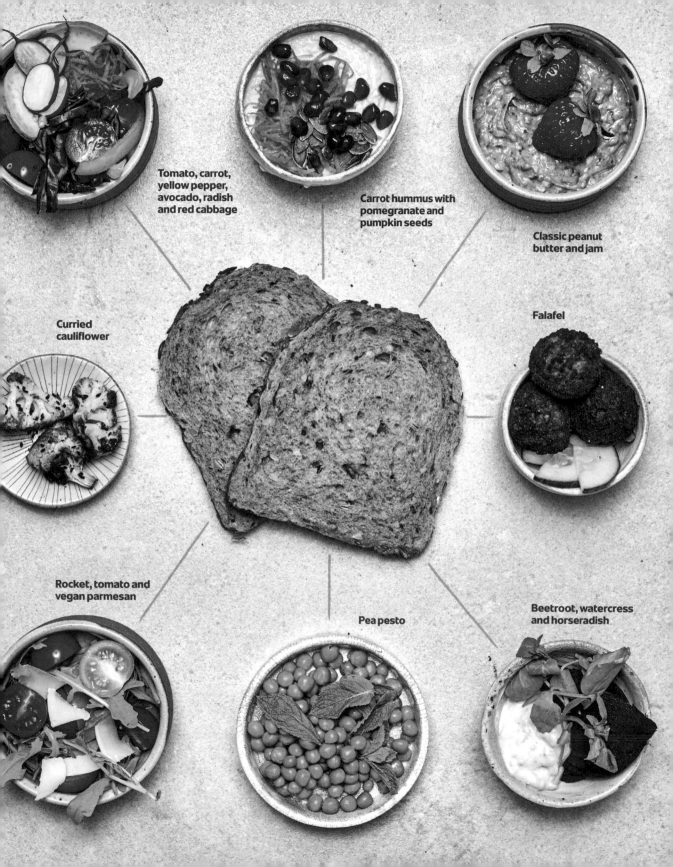

Tomato, carrot, yellow pepper, avocado, radish and red cabbage

Carrot hummus with pomegranate and pumpkin seeds

Classic peanut butter and jam

Curried cauliflower

Falafel

Rocket, tomato and vegan parmesan

Pea pesto

Beetroot, watercress and horseradish

DIY POT NOODLES

Makes 4 portions

4 small nests of instant wholegrain rice noodles

A sheet of nori, shredded

1 small courgette, cut into matchsticks

1 small carrot, cut into matchsticks

1 red pepper, finely sliced

4 large leaves of kale or similar, finely shredded

4 spring onions

4 mushrooms

4 tbsp frozen peas

For the sauce

4 tbsp miso paste

4 tbsp tamari or light soy sauce

2 garlic cloves

10g piece of ginger, grated

½ tsp ground turmeric

½ tsp Chinese 5 spice

If you are looking for a quick lunchtime option, this DIY Pot Noodles recipe fits the bill. I've found the best noodles to use are instant wholegrain rice noodles because they soften in the right time. You can use whatever vegetables you have to hand. For example, one pack of stir-fry veg can easily feed four. Aim to get as many types of veggies and colours as you can into yours.

Take 4 large jars or round screw-top Tupperware. Layer them up with the noodles on the bottom, followed by the seaweed and vegetables. Mix all the sauce ingredients together and spoon over the vegetables. Seal until ready to cook.

When you are ready to cook the noodles, boil a kettle. Add the freshly boiled water to around halfway up the jar if you want it fairly dry, to the top if you want it soupier. Leave to stand for around 3 minutes, then give it a good stir with chopsticks, pulling the noodles up from the base to make sure they are cooked.

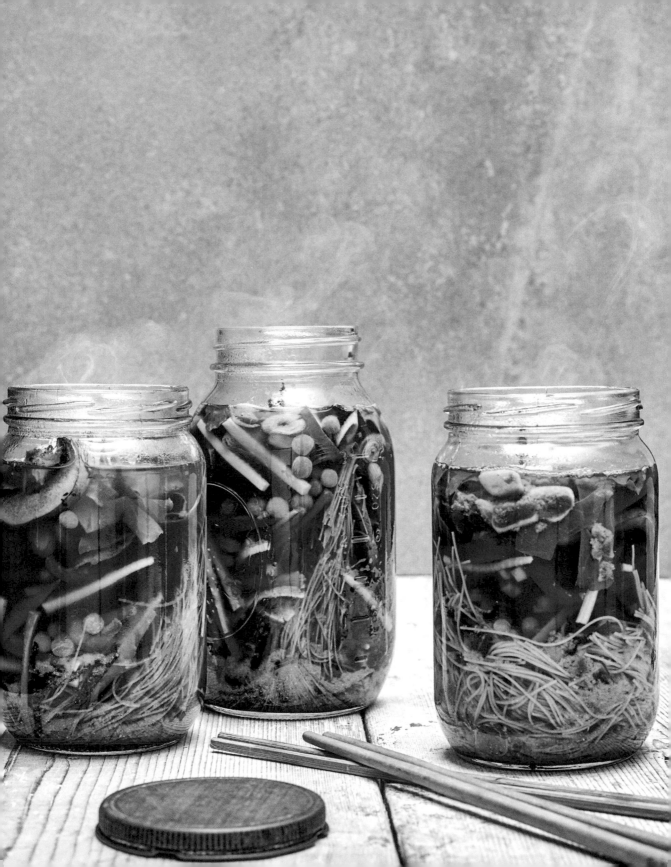

WINTER VEGETABLE AND BARLEY SOUP

Makes 4–6 portions

1 tbsp olive oil (or use no-oil sautéeing method)

1 onion, finely diced

2 sticks celery, finely diced

700g vegetables, unpeeled, if possible, and diced – select at least 3 from: carrots, pumpkin, squash, celeriac, beetroot, swede, parsnip, turnip, kohlrabi

A bouquet garni of 2 sprigs rosemary, 2 sprigs parsley and 2 bay leaves

1 tsp dried oregano

4 garlic cloves, lightly crushed

100g pearled barley

1.2 litres vegetable stock

1 tsp Marmite or alternative yeast extract (optional)

150g cavolo nero, kale, Savoy cabbage or similar, shredded

Salt and pepper

This hearty soup is perfect for colder months when you need something filling and nutritious to power you through the afternoon. This recipe is very versatile and can made using any root veg you have at home. I have listed a few options on the left for veggie ideas you can add or swap depending on what's in your fridge.

If using the oil, heat it in a large saucepan or casserole. Add the onion, celery and all the vegetables and sauté gently, stirring regularly, until starting to caramelise slightly around the edges. If not using the oil, add all the vegetables to the saucepan with 2 tbsp water. Cook over a low heat, stirring very regularly, and add more water at intervals until everything is starting to brown.

Add the bouquet garni, oregano and garlic to the pan along with the pearled barley. Season with salt and pepper and add the vegetable stock and the Marmite or yeast extract, if using. Bring to the boil, then reduce the heat to a simmer and partially cover. Simmer gently for around 30 minutes until the vegetables are well on their way to being tender. Add the kale or cabbage to the pot and push down into the liquid. Add a little more stock or water if necessary – it should be quite a thick, hearty soup. Continue to simmer for another 30 minutes until the greens are completely wilted down, the vegetables are tender and breaking up, and the barley is cooked through. Check for seasoning and serve.

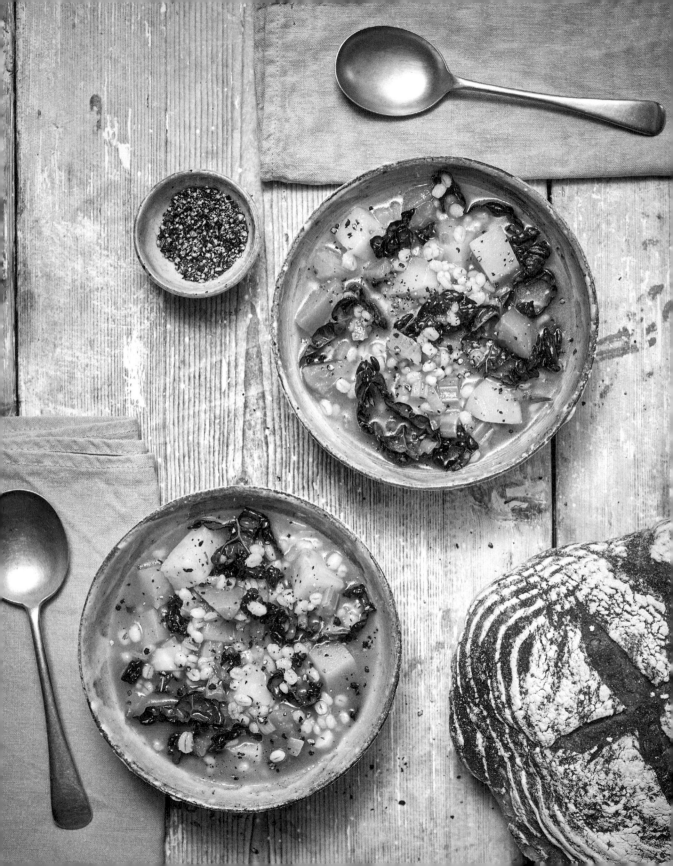

CAESAR SALAD

Makes 4 portions

For the croutons

2 tsp vegan balsamic vinegar

1 tsp dried mixed herbs

100g wholegrain bread, cut into cubes

Salt and pepper

For the dressing

300g silken tofu

1 tsp garlic powder

1 tbsp mustard

1 tbsp capers

1 tbsp tamari

Juice of ½ lemon

For the salad

1 garlic clove, cut in half

1 large head Cos or 2 Romaine lettuces

4 spring onions, sliced

150g cavolo nero, kale, Savoy cabbage or similar

Grated vegan parmesan (optional)

4 slices of cooked tofu bacon, crumbled (see page 205)

My Caesar salad is a plant-based take on the classic dish and has an incredibly creamy oil-free dressing that is very adaptable and so simple to make. It can easily perk up any salad you have lingering in the fridge.

First make the croutons. Preheat your oven to 200°C/400°F/gas mark 6. Put 2 tbsp water in a large bowl and add the balsamic vinegar and herbs. Season with salt and pepper, then add the bread cubes and toss to coat. Arrange over a baking tray and bake in the oven for around 10 minutes until crisp.

Make the dressing by putting all the ingredients in a food processor with plenty of seasoning and blending until smooth. Leave to stand while you prepare the salad.

Take a salad bowl and rub the inside of it with the garlic. Roughly tear up the lettuce and add to the bowl with the spring onions. Sprinkle the kale with salt and massage with your hands until it softens, then shred and add to the bowl.

Add a few tablespoons of the dressing and vegan parmesan, if using, and toss thoroughly. Sprinkle over the croutons and tofu bacon bits and serve.

DINNER

What's for dinner?

If your household is anything like mine and this question is always on everyone's lips, then cooking can feel like a chore. It doesn't need to be! Here, I have detailed some of my favourite go-to plant-based dishes for dinner and they are very simple and quick to make! These include some of my best swaps for meat-based choices and dishes loaded with vegetables, legumes and wholegrains. I've also included my go-to tomato sauce that can be transformed into curry, chilli or soup.

TOMATO SAUCE, VARIOUS WAYS

Makes 4 portions

The basic recipe

1 tbsp olive oil (optional)

1 onion, very finely chopped

2 garlic cloves, finely chopped

1 tsp dried oregano

2 bay leaves

2 x 400g tins tomatoes

A pinch of ground cinnamon

Salt and pepper

Tomato sauce makes the perfect base for a host of dishes. Tomatoes are packed full of the antioxidant lycopene, as well as vitamin C, potassium, folate and vitamin K. This simple dish, which starts with oregano and bay leaves in the basic recipe, means you will never have to turn to a ready-made jar of tomato sauce again. Build on your base to make warming curries, chillis and soups.

If using the oil, heat it in a casserole or saucepan and sauté the onion until soft and translucent. If not using oil, sauté the onion in water – add a tablespoon to start with and keep an eye on it, adding a little more water as necessary, until the onion is tender.

Add the garlic and cook for a further 2 minutes, then add the oregano, bay leaves and tomatoes, along with 200ml water (use the water to swill out the tins and add to the sauce). Season with plenty of salt and pepper, then bring to the boil, reduce the heat and cover. Simmer for 20 minutes. Taste – if the sauce is too acidic, add a pinch of cinnamon, this will help bring out the sweetness of the tomatoes. Continue to simmer, this time uncovered until the sauce is well reduced. Taste again and adjust the seasoning if necessary.

Top tip – I also love adding a spoonful of miso paste, harissa paste or smoked paprika to my tomato sauce before simmering to bring the sauce to life, depending on the desired flavour that day. Let me know your favourite flavour combos!

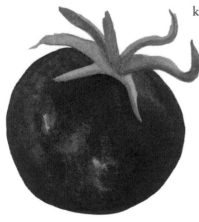

FROM FRESH

Make the sauce using 1kg fresh tomatoes. Peel the tomatoes by coring and putting a cross on the base of each one with a sharp knife, cover with freshly boiled water for 15 seconds then drain – the skins should peel off easily. Roughly chop and add to the sauce. Alternatively, put whole tomatoes in a high-powered blender and blitz until smooth. Add to the onion and just bring to the boil, reduce the heat and simmer uncovered until the sauce has reduced. Add the basil as in the Summer variation below.

SUMMER

Add 3–4 whole basil leaves 5 minutes from the end of cooking – this will imbue the sauce with the flavour and aroma of the basil.

WINTER

For a richer, very robust sauce good for winter and meaty vegetables like aubergines, add 100ml red wine before you add the tomatoes. Reduce the red wine by half and add a sprig or two of thyme to the sauce as well.

AS A BASE FOR A CHILLI

Swap the white onion for red and add a red or green pepper when sautéeing. Add 1 tbsp chipotle sauce (or similar hot sauce), 1 tsp each of ground cumin and coriander and ½ tsp ground cinnamon to the tomatoes along with the herbs. When the sauce has cooked for 20 minutes add 2 x 400g tins beans (black or pinto are good) and 150g sweetcorn. Serve with plenty of coriander.

AS A BASE FOR A CURRY

Add your favourite curry paste or blend along with the garlic and 2 tbsp finely chopped coriander stems or some ground turmeric, omitting the herbs. Add the tomatoes and simmer as before. Blanch any vegetables before adding to the sauce and finish with a little coconut milk and plenty of chopped coriander.

AS A BASE FOR A SOUP

Add a litre of vegetable stock or a mixture of vegetable stock and coconut milk along with the tomatoes. You can also add other vegetables. Add 200g squash or carrots along with the garlic, as well as 50g well-rinsed red lentils, then simmer in the vegetable stock until the vegetables are tender before adding the tomatoes. Simmer for a further 20 minutes, then blitz until smooth.

VEGAN BOLOGNESE

Makes 4 portions

1 tbsp olive oil (if using oil)

1 onion, finely chopped

1 small carrot, finely chopped

1 stick celery, finely chopped

1 small aubergine, finely diced

100g mushrooms, finely diced

4 garlic cloves, finely chopped

1 tsp dried oregano

1 bay leaf

100ml red wine (optional, can add more stock instead)

400g tin tomatoes

200ml mushroom or vegetable stock

Salt and pepper

To serve

500g wholemeal spaghetti or other type of pasta

Vegan parmesan (optional)

This hearty and rich dish is the perfect alternative to a meat-based version with mushrooms and aubergines for texture and red wine for extra flavour – it hits the spot every time! Some of these veggies can be substituted with Quorn® or soya mince but these products can sometimes be processed, so use natural alternatives where you can.

If using the oil, heat it in a large casserole or saucepan. Add the onion, carrot, celery, aubergine and mushrooms and sauté, stirring regularly. If not using oil, add a little water to the pan at the same time. Sauté in the same way, stirring regularly. Eventually the vegetables will collapse down to around half their original volume and any liquid they have given out will evaporate off. At this point, increase the heat and allow to brown.

Add the garlic and cook for a further couple of minutes, then stir in the herbs and red wine. Bring to the boil and bubble until most of the wine has evaporated, then add the tomatoes and stock. Season with salt and pepper.

Leave to simmer for around 30 minutes until the sauce has reduced down and smells rich and savoury.

Cook the pasta in plenty of boiling, salted water until al dente. Serve the pasta with the sauce spooned over and a little vegan parmesan, if using.

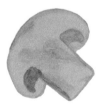

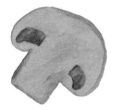

HOW TO MAKE LASAGNE

Use either a portion of Bolognese (opposite) or tomato sauce (see page 220) and a portion of mac-n-cheese sauce (see page 224) to make a lasagne. Thin the mac-n-cheese sauce down a little more with another 100ml plant-based milk. Layer the Bolognese up with a few tablespoons of the mac-n-cheese sauce and lasagne, topping with more mac-n-cheese sauce and finally breadcrumbs mixed with basil. You can add any other vegetables to this – you can grill vegetables or buy jars of grilled vegetables in brine (look for courgettes, peppers, aubergines and artichokes) and add cherry tomatoes or sliced tomatoes to each layer. Bake in the oven at 200°C/400°F/gas mark 6 for 35–45 minutes.

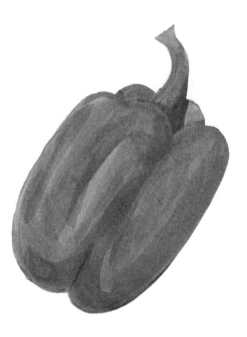

MAC-N-CHEESE

Makes 4 portions

500g bag macaroni

For the sauce

100g cashew nuts

1 large carrot, cut into chunks

1 medium potato, cut into chunks

1 onion, roughly chopped

1 celery stick roughly chopped

150g sweet potato or butternut squash, cut into chunks

3 garlic cloves, roughly chopped

1 tsp dried oregano

1 tsp mustard powder

2 tbsp nutritional yeast (optional)

200ml plant-based milk

If baking

150g cherry tomatoes

50g wholemeal breadcrumbs

A few basil leaves, finely chopped (optional)

50g vegan cheese (optional)

To serve (optional)

Vegan parmesan

Amazingly creamy and nutty, this dish will always leave you satisfied. There are several ways to make it but I use cashew nuts and boil them along with the veggies to save time, heat, water and washing up. Win–win! This is blended, so there is no need to peel the sweet potato, squash or carrot – in fact, a lot of nutrients are in the skin – but do wash them thoroughly first.

This recipe includes nutritional yeast, which is a great source of B vitamins (though not B12) and it is also a complete protein. I love the flavour, which is very cheesy, so can give any dish a parmesan-style kick.

Preheat the oven to 200°C/400°F/gas mark 6. Put the cashew nuts in a saucepan of water and bring to the boil. Boil fiercely for 5 minutes, then add all the vegetables and the garlic. Continue to simmer for at least 10 minutes until all the vegetables are very tender.

Drain and transfer to a blender. Add all the remaining sauce ingredients and season with salt. Blend until smooth.

Bring a large pot of water to the boil and a handful of salt. Add the macaroni and cook according to the packet instructions. Drain and mix with the vegetable sauce. If you like, sprinkle with vegan parmesan.

The macaroni cheese can be eaten like this or you can bake in the oven. If you are doing this, transfer to an ovenproof dish and stir through the tomatoes. Mix the breadcrumbs with the basil and vegan cheese, if using, then bake for around 25 minutes until it is piping hot and bubbling.

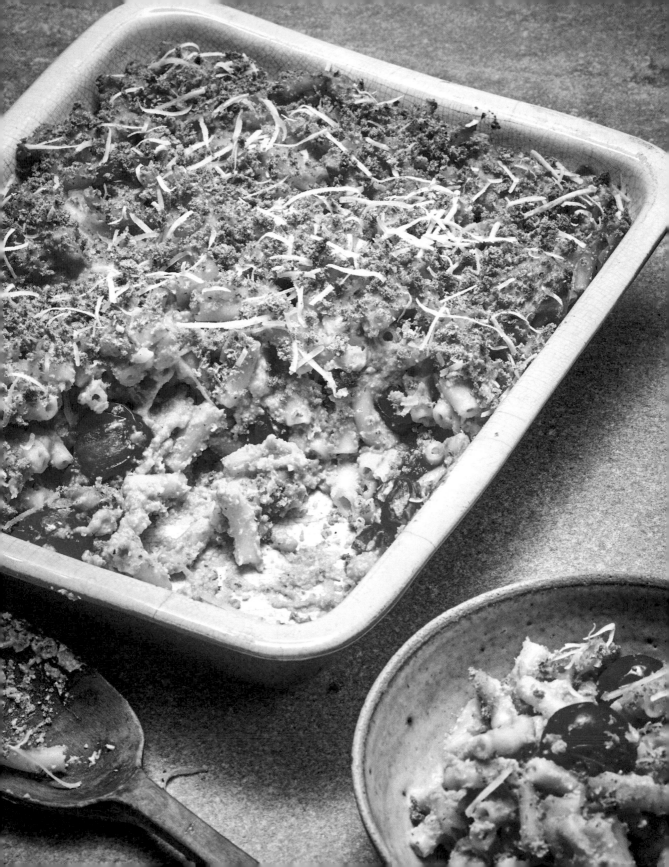

MUSHROOM CASSEROLE WITH WHITE BEAN MASH

Makes 4 portions

2 tsp olive oil (optional)

3 large carrots, cut into chunks

12 button onions or shallots, peeled

500g chestnut mushrooms, halved

2 garlic cloves, crushed

2 large sprigs thyme or dried thyme

2 bay leaves

200ml red wine (optional, otherwise just add more stock)

400ml mushroom stock

2 tsp cornflour or arrowroot (optional)

Salt and pepper

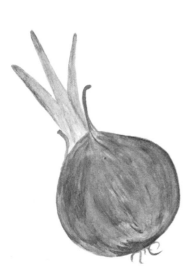

Mushrooms are a powerhouse of vitamins, minerals and fibre and offer a host of health benefits. This is one of my go-to recipes when I am craving something filling on a cold day. I've switched out mashed potatoes for cannellini or butter beans, which have a rich and creamy texture and are a great source of macronutrients for us and for our gut microbiome.

If using oil, heat a teaspoon of the olive oil in a large casserole. Add the carrots and onions and sauté, stirring regularly, until they have taken on some colour. If not using the oil, add a tablespoon of water at the beginning of the cooking process and keep adding a little more until the same result is achieved. Remove the onions and carrots from the pan and follow the same procedure with the mushrooms, using either the remaining oil or more water. When you can see that the amount of liquid in the casserole is increasing (it will do so as the mushrooms reduce in volume), let it evaporate off and add the garlic. Cook for a couple more minutes, stirring constantly.

Add the thyme and bay leaves and return the onions and carrots to the casserole. Pour over the wine and season with salt and pepper. Bring to the boil and allow the wine to reduce down by half, then add the stock. Return to the boil, then turn down to a simmer and cover. Cook for around 25 minutes, by which point the vegetables should be tender. If not, cook for a little longer.

If you want a thicker, glossy sauce, use the cornflour or arrowroot. Blend with a little cold water and stir into the casserole after it has cooked for around 25 minutes. Stir over a medium heat until the sauce thickens.

For the mash

75ml plant-based milk

3 garlic cloves, thinly sliced

2 x 400g tins cannellini or butter beans

A squeeze of lemon juice

2 tbsp finely chopped parsley

While the casserole is cooking, make the mash. Heat the plant-based milk and garlic in a saucepan until the garlic is tender. Transfer to a blender or food processor and blitz until smooth. Pour the beans and their liquid into a saucepan and heat through. When piping hot, strain, return to the saucepan with the milk and garlic mixture and roughly purée – you want some texture. Season with a squeeze of lemon juice, salt and pepper, then stir in the the chopped parsley. Serve alongside the mushroom casserole.

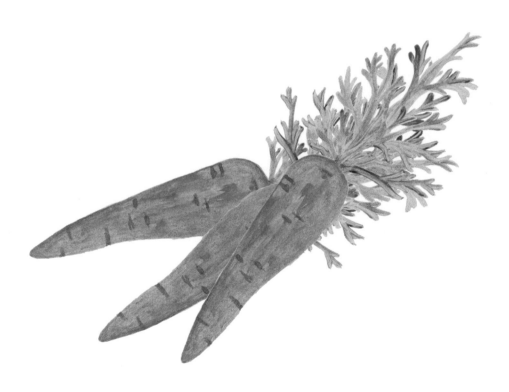

PASTA WITH GREENS AND PESTO

Makes 4 portions

500g wholemeal spaghetti

1 large courgette, coarsely grated

100g baby spinach

Salt

For the pesto

50g nuts – pine nuts, cashew nuts and almonds are all good

Zest and juice of 1 lemon

A large bunch of basil

1 garlic clove

2 tbsp nutritional yeast (optional)

To serve

Vegan parmesan (optional)

This is super-easy and quick to make and once you have made your own home-made pesto, you will never look back. I've made the nutritional yeast optional as the recipe doesn't necessarily need it but if you are a fan, add some in for additional flavour.

First make the pesto. Put the nuts into a food processor and pulse until they are the texture of coarse breadcrumbs. Add the lemon zest and juice, the basil and the garlic clove. Pulse, pushing down regularly, until you have a thick, slightly grainy paste, adding a little water to thin if it is proving reluctant to break down.

Bring a large pot of water to the boil. When it is at a fast rolling boil, add a tablespoon of salt and the pasta. Cook until it is almost done, then add the courgette and spinach. Leave to wilt for a minute. Ladle off some of the cooking liquid, then drain the pasta and greens.

Return to the saucepan and add the pesto and some of the cooking liquid – the starches in the liquid will help make the sauce creamy.

Make sure everything is piping hot and serve with a grating of vegan parmesan, if using.

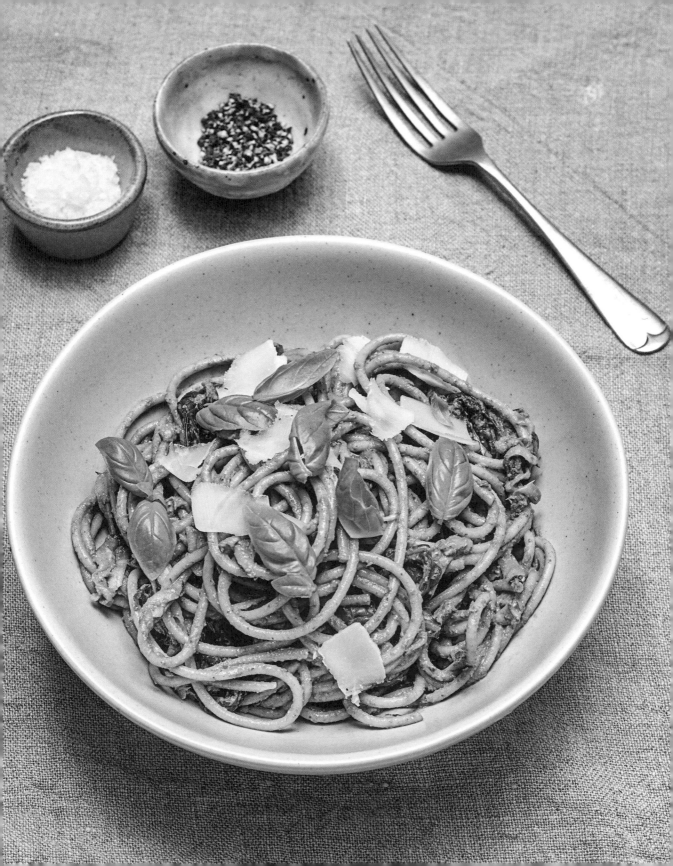

BAKED POTATOES

Makes 4 portions

4 potatoes or sweet potatoes

A little salt

You can't go wrong with baked potatoes and these plant-based fillings are simple and easy to make. My favourite is the creamy garlic mushrooms and spinach. Enjoy!

To bake the potatoes, preheat your oven to 180°C/350°F/gas mark 4. Pierce the potatoes all over with a fork or skewer, then score a deep cross on the top. Sprinkle with salt. Bake regular potatoes in the oven for just over an hour, sweet potatoes take less time – around 45 minutes.

BAKED BEANS

Perhaps with some smoked, marinated tofu stirred through (see page 205).

STEAMED BROCCOLI AND SPRING ONIONS WITH VEGAN CHEESE SAUCE

Steam the broccoli and spring onions until tender then roughly chop the spring onions. Divide between the baked potatoes and spoon over some vegan cheese sauce (use the sauce from the Mac-n-cheese – see page 224).

WHITE BEANS WITH CHIPOTLE SAUCE

Blitz 100g silken tofu with 1 tbsp chipotle paste, 1 tsp garlic powder and juice of ½ lime. Heat the 2 tins of beans, then drain, roughly mash and mix with a few sliced spring onions, more lime juice and plenty of chopped coriander. Stir a couple of tablespoons of the chipotle sauce through and spoon into the centre of the potatoes. Drizzle over a little more of the sauce.

CREAMY GARLIC MUSHROOMS AND SPINACH

Take 400g of any type of mushrooms and slice thinly. If using oil, add to a sauté pan and sauté the mushrooms with 1 finely sliced shallot. If not using the oil, add a little water and sauté until the mushrooms start giving out water, then continue cooking until the liquid evaporates and they brown. Add 2 crushed garlic cloves and 4 cubes of frozen spinach along with 2 tbsp vegan cream. Spoon into the baked potatoes and add lots of finely chopped parsley and a squeeze of lemon juice.

CREAMY COLESLAW

Shred half a white cabbage, a carrot and a bunch of spring onions. Sprinkle with salt and leave to stand in a colander for 30 minutes. For the cashew cream, boil 100g cashew nuts in water for 15 minutes or until soft, then blitz in a blender with 100ml water, 2 tsp cider vinegar, 1 tsp garlic powder and 1 tsp maple syrup. Toss the vegetables in the sauce and sprinkle with sesame seeds.

BROWN RICE AND LENTILS (KITCHIRI)

Makes 4–6 portions

1 tsp mustard seeds

1 tsp cumin seeds

1 small can (160ml) coconut cream

25g piece ginger, grated

3 garlic cloves, crushed

1 onion, finely sliced

1 large carrot, coarsely grated

1 tsp ground turmeric

½ tsp ground cinnamon

Stems from a bunch of coriander, finely chopped

200g brown basmati rice

50g lentils, soaked overnight unless red lentils

1 litre vegetable stock or water

200g frozen peas

Salt and pepper

To serve

Leaves from a bunch of coriander

Green chillies, finely chopped

Lemon or lime wedges

Nourish your body with this delicious recipe. Kitchiri is one of the staple healing foods in Ayurveda because it is balancing, immune-boosting and easy to digest. It is traditionally a simple dish and I have made it extra wholesome with brown rice, more veggies and a fraction of the oil and fat content of the traditional version.

Heat the mustard and cumin seeds in a large saucepan or casserole until they start to pop, then add the 2 tbsp of the coconut cream, the ginger, garlic, onion, carrot and spices. Stir to combine so the vegetables look as though they are coated with a thick, brightly coloured paste. Cook for 2 minutes, then add the coriander stems, rice, lentils and stock. Season with salt and pepper, stir, and bring to the boil. Reduce the heat, cover, and leave to simmer for around 20 minutes until the rice and lentils are cooked through. Add the peas and taste. If you think it could be sweeter, add the remaining coconut cream. Simmer until the peas are tender, adding extra water if it appears to be drying out. Serve with coriander leaves, green chillies and lemon or lime wedges

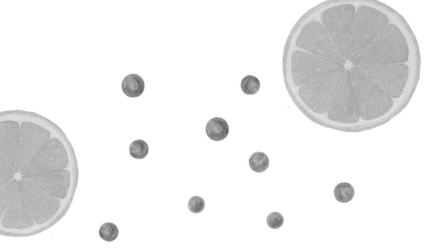

PULLED JACKFRUIT BURGER WITH COLESLAW

Makes 4 portions

For the jackfruit

2 tins young or unripe jackfruit, drained

1 tbsp olive oil (optional)

For the BBQ sauce

300ml passata

1 tsp molasses or black treacle

1 tbsp maple syrup

2 tsp cider vinegar

1 tbsp soy sauce

1 tsp garlic powder

1 garlic clove, grated

1 tsp dried oregano

A few dashes of hot sauce

½ onion, studded with 5 cloves

A few drops of liquid smoke

Salt and pepper

For the coleslaw

½ small white or Savoy cabbage, finely shredded

1 carrot, coarsely grated

1 onion, finely sliced

A small bunch of coriander

Zest and juice of 1 lime

To serve

4 wholemeal vegan burger buns

4 large floppy green lettuce leaves

Sliced gherkins

4 slices tomato

Jackfruit is a member of the fig family and is grown on trees. It has a sweet and fruity flavour and is fantastically stringy, so it is an ideal swap for meat like pulled pork or shredded chicken. I've grilled the jackfruit here to give it some char and more depth of flavour but this step can be missed out.

If you add chipotle to this, it would also make a great filling for tacos. Here, I've made my BBQ sauce from scratch but if you are short of time, you may want to use a shop-bought option instead.

First make the BBQ sauce. Put all the ingredients except the liquid smoke into a saucepan and season with salt and pepper. Bring to the boil, then reduce the heat to a simmer. Continue to cook until the sauce is well reduced and thick – it should be thick enough that it leaves a trail on the base of the pan when you scrape a spoon across it. When then sauce is ready, remove from the heat and discard the onion and cloves.

Next make the coleslaw. Sprinkle the cabbage, carrot and onion with salt and leave to stand in a colander for 30 minutes. Drain and toss with the coriander, lime zest and juice. Season with a little more salt and pepper if necessary. Set aside.

Heat a non-stick pan or griddle. Drain your jackfruit and toss in the olive oil, if using. Season with salt. Arrange on your pan or griddle and cook on each side until lightly charred. Remove and set aside to cool. When the jackfruit is cool enough to handle, pull away the strands from the core and shred, discarding the core and any seeds.

Add the jackfruit to the BBQ sauce and simmer. Add a few drops of liquid smoke for a smokier flavour.

Assemble each burger by lightly toasting the buns, then layering with lettuce, sliced gherkins, tomato, jackfruit and coleslaw.

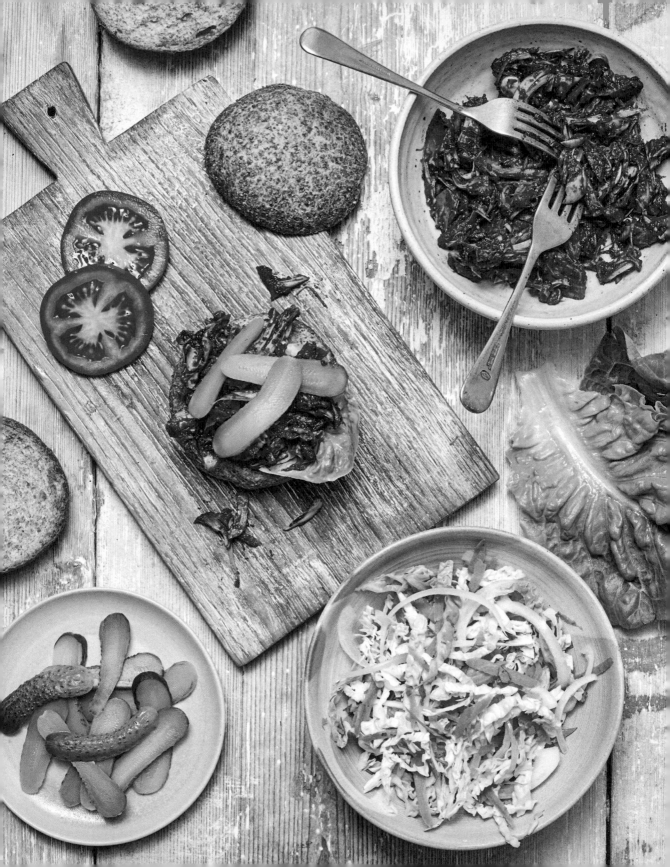

SHEPHERDLESS PIE

Makes 4 portions

1 tbsp olive oil (optional)

1 onion, finely chopped

1 stick celery, finely chopped

300g selection of root veg, use what you have: carrot, beetroot, parsnip, celeriac, diced

2 garlic cloves, finely chopped

400g cooked brown lentils

1 sprig rosemary, finely chopped (or dried herbs)

1 sprig thyme, finely chopped (or dried herbs)

1 tbsp mustard ketchup

1 tsp Dijon mustard

100ml red wine (optional)

300ml vegetable stock

For the mash

700g potatoes, peeled and chopped

3 garlic cloves, unpeeled

75ml plant-based milk

25g breadcrumbs

A small bunch of parsley

This is one of my favourite recipes. My family loves this take on the classic comfort food and always ask for seconds. I haven't put any green vegetables in but they can be added easily. This is best served with a large bowl of green peas.

If using oil, heat it in a large saucepan. Add the onion, celery and selection of vegetables and sauté until lightly browned. If not using oil, add all the vegetables to the saucepan with 1–2 tbsp water, and sauté, adding more water if it becomes too dry, until the vegetables are lightly browned.

Add the garlic and cook for a further couple of minutes, then stir in the lentils, herbs, mustard ketchup and Dijon mustard. Pour in the red wine and bring to the boil. Allow the wine to boil away almost completely, then add the vegetable stock. Continue to simmer until the vegetables are tender.

While the base is cooking, boil the potatoes in plenty of salted water with the garlic until tender. Drain thoroughly and squish the garlic out of its skins. Add to the potatoes with the plant-based milk and mash thoroughly.

Preheat the oven to 200°C/400°F/gas mark 6. Arrange the vegetables in the base of an ovenproof dish, then top with the mashed potatoes. Mix the breadcrumbs and parsley together and sprinkle over the potatoes. Bake in the preheated oven for around 30 minutes until lightly speckled brown and bubbling.

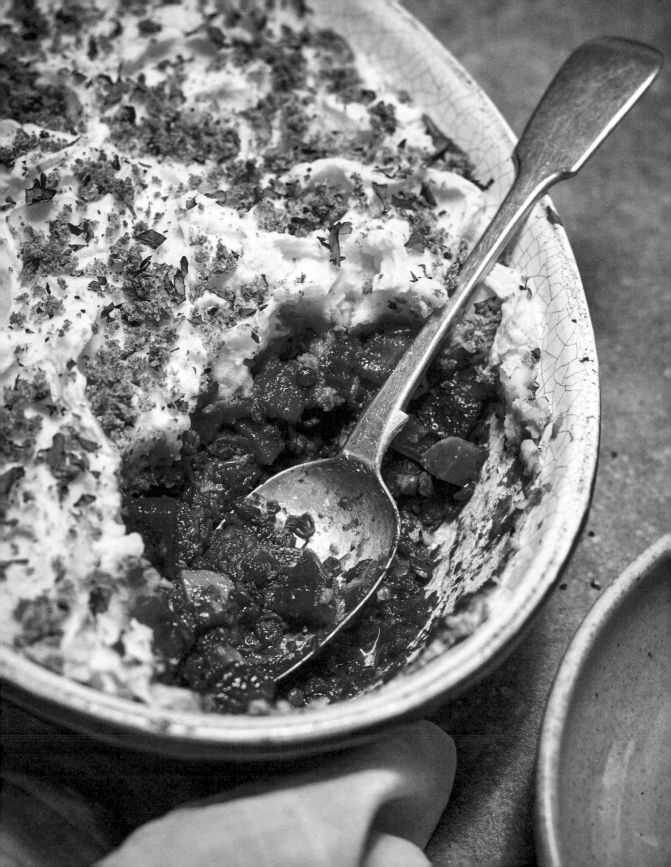

SWEET AND SOUR TOFU

Makes 4 portions

For the tofu

1 block of firm or extra firm tofu, pressed

2 tbsp arrowroot

½ tsp chilli powder (optional)

For the sweet and sour sauce

50ml soy sauce

25ml rice wine vinegar

50ml pineapple juice

1 tbsp apricot jam

2 tsp maple or date syrup

½ tsp Chinese 5 spice

½ tsp garlic powder

½ tsp chilli powder

1 tsp cornflour

For the stir-fry

2 tsp sesame oil (optional)

1 red pepper, cut into chunks

100g mange tout or asparagus tips or sprouting broccoli spears – blanch them first, or slice them lengthways

100g baby corn

2 garlic cloves, finely chopped

15g piece ginger, finely chopped (or a frozen cube)

To serve

3 spring onions, halved lengthways and shredded

A few sprigs coriander

A few drops of sesame oil and/or 1 tsp sesame seeds (optional)

Brown rice or noodles

This plant-based version of the classic Chinese meal has that irresistible tangy sweet-and-sour flavour. I find that baking the tofu in the oven first is the easiest way to get it nice and crispy if you are cooking without oil.

First bake the tofu. Preheat the oven to 200°C/400°F/gas mark 6 and line a baking tray with baking parchment. Cut the tofu into chunks and pat dry. Mix the arrowroot with the chilli powder, if using, and a little salt and toss in the tofu chunks, making sure they are evenly coated. Arrange on a baking tray, making sure they are not touching, then bake for 15–20 minutes until crisp and brown.

Whisk together all the sweet and sour sauce ingredients except the cornflour and set aside.

Heat a wok and add the oil, if using. When the air above is shimmering, add the the vegetables, garlic and ginger and stir-fry for 2–3 minutes. If not using the oil, use 1 tbsp water instead, adding a little more after a couple of minutes if necessary.

Pour in the sauce and simmer for 2–3 minutes until it looks syrupy, then mix the cornflour with a little water and add to the wok, stirring constantly until the sauce has thickened slightly and is glossy. Add the tofu and simmer for a further minute, then serve sprinkled with the spring onions, coriander and sesame oil or seeds, if using.

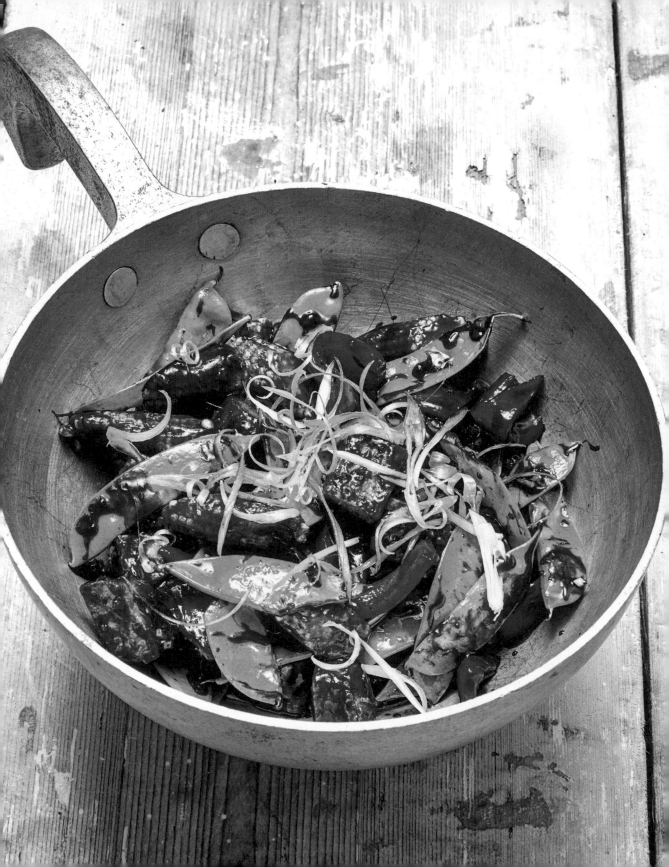

VEGETABLE TIKKA MASALA

Makes 4–6 portions

2 tsp olive oil (optional)

1 large onion, finely chopped

4 garlic cloves, crushed

25g piece ginger, crushed

1 tbsp medium curry powder

1 tsp ground cumin

1 tsp ground turmeric

1 tbsp tomato purée

300g piece butternut squash, cut into large chunks – peeled or unpeeled is fine

½ cauliflower, cut into florets

1 x 400g tin tomatoes

1 x 400g tin coconut milk

1 x 400g tin chickpeas

A squeeze of lemon (optional)

Salt and pepper

To serve

Coriander

Brown rice

I love making curries and this one is bursting with flavour. I've used curry powder here instead of individual spices, as it would make the ingredients list very long but I would recommended getting a blend for tikka masala or a deep red medium curry powder (not the milder yellow one).

If using the oil, heat it in a large casserole or saucepan and add the onion. If not using the oil, add 2 tbsp water. Sauté the onion until soft and translucent, stirring regularly and adding a little more water if necessary. Add the garlic, ginger, curry powder, cumin, turmeric and tomato purée. Continue to stir until the onion is completely coated, adding more water if it looks dry.

Add the squash and cauliflower. Turn over gently in the sauce until covered, then add the tomatoes, coconut milk and chickpeas. Season with plenty of salt and pepper. Bring to the boil, then treduce the heat and simmer, uncovered, until the vegetables are tender and the sauce has thickened. Taste and add a squeeze of lemon juice and more seasoning if necessary.

Serve garnished with plenty of coriander, and some brown rice on the side.

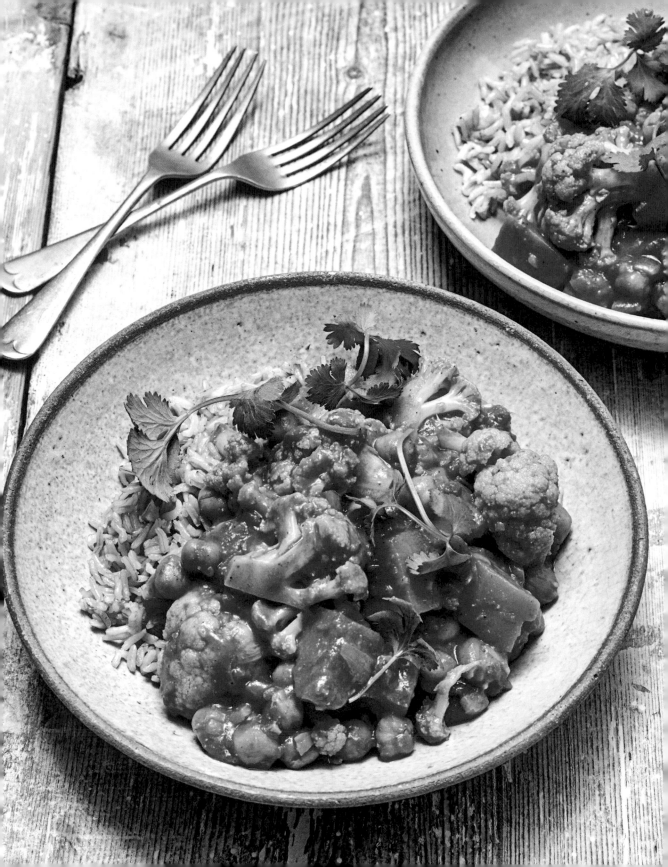

SALADS

The aim of my salads is to make them as colourful and varied as possible. I have listed groups of ingredients here as examples but when you make your own, try to include at least four veggies, a grain and a protein.

GREENS

Shredded lettuce
Rocket, spinach
Chinese cabbage
Very finely shredded kale
or green cabbage

OTHER VEGETABLES

Coarsely grated carrot
Celeriac
Kohlrabi
Beetroot
Shredded red cabbage
Courgette
Green beans, blanched
Any coloured peppers, finely sliced
Sliced radishes
Baby corn or sweetcorn
Lightly steamed broccoli
Sweetcorn
Tomatoes
Cucumber

BEANS

Black beans
Chickpeas
Puy lentils
Brown lentils
Butter beans

GRAINS

Quinoa
Brown or wild rice
Spelt
Barley
Buckwheat
Wholemeal couscous
Freekeh

FLAVOURS

Coriander
Parsley
Oregano
Chillies
Limes
Lemons
Spring onions
Red onions
Microleaves, such as basil
Methi

TOPPING

Cashew cream sauce
(see Creamy Coleslaw, page 230)

SEEDS AND NUTS

Pumpkin
Sunflower
Linseed
Sesame
Toasted almonds
Pecans
Walnuts
Hazelnuts

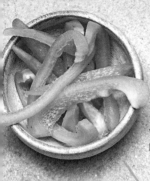

Yellow pepper

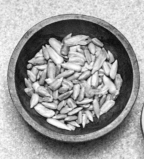

Sunflower (left) and pumpkin seeds

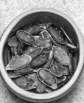

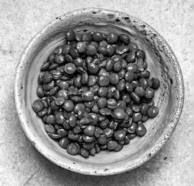

Brown lentils

Cucumber

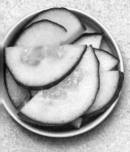

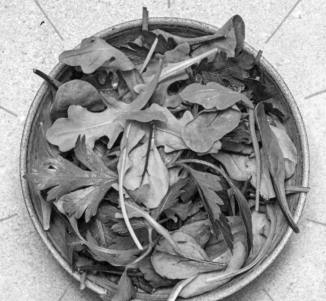

Chickpeas

Flaked almonds

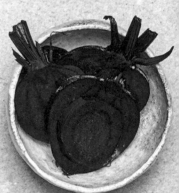

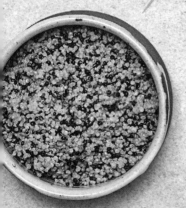

Beetroot

Quinoa

Tomatoes

Radishes

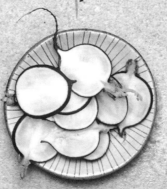

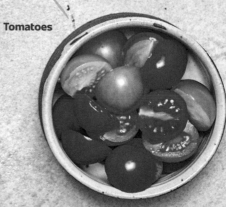

WINTER SALAD

Divide 300g cooked brown rice or pearled barley between 4 bowls. Strip the leaves from a large bunch of kale. Put in a bowl with a pinch of salt and massage the kale until the texture changes – it should soften without wilting. Roughly chop and divide between 4 bowls, placing on top of the brown rice. Coarsely grate a carrot and place next to the kale. Grate a beetroot and mix with a quarter of a red cabbage and place next to the carrot. Divide 100g cooked green lentils between the bowls. Mix together 1 tbsp cider vinegar, ½ tsp mustard and the juice of ½ orange. Drizzle this over the bowls. Sprinkle over 2 shredded spring onions and some finely chopped parsley and 2 tbsp chopped hazelnuts.

SPICY SWEETCORN AND BLACK BEAN SALAD

Divide 300g cooked quinoa or brown rice between 4 bowls. Split a well washed bag of spinach, a drained and well rinsed 400g tin of black or pinto beans, 300g cooked sweetcorn, 4 chopped tomatoes and 8 slices of avocado between the bowls. Slice a red onion and toss in the juice of 1 lime and scatter over along with lots of coriander and fresh or pickled jalapeños. (Add a cashew cream sauce with chipotle if you like.)

COURGETTE, POMEGRANATE AND ALMOND SALAD

Divide 300g wholemeal couscous between 4 bowls. Squeeze the juice of ½ orange and a lemon over it. Finely chop small bunches of mint, parsley and coriander and fork through the couscous. With a potato peeler, cut a courgette into thin ribbons and toss with salt, ½ tsp dried oregano and the juice of 1 lemon. Add this to the bowls. Add 1 grated carrot, 2 grated turnips, 100g rocket and 200g blanched green beans. Drizzle with a dressing made from 2 tbsp tahini, 1 tsp date syrup and the juice of 1 lemon. Top with the seeds from half a pomegranate and 2 tbsp toasted almonds.

You can change this up by replacing the tahini with harissa in the dressing.

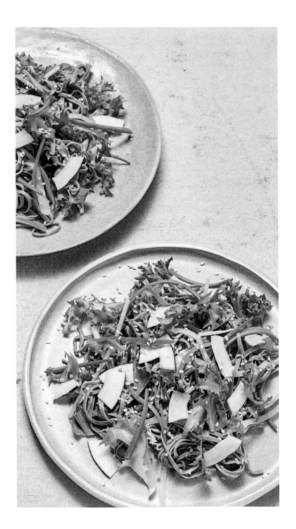

MISO NOODLE SALAD

Toss buckwheat noodles in a few drops of sesame oil and divide between 4 bowls. Make a dressing with 2 tbsp tamari, 1 tbsp miso paste, 1 tbsp rice vinegar, juice of ½ lemon, 1 crushed garlic clove, 10g grated ginger and 1 tsp maple syrup. Add 1 shredded carrot, shredded radish or daikon and lots of mustard salad greens, such as mizuna, to the noodles. Slice 2 spring onions and add those too. Shred some fresh coconut and sprinkle over with some sesame seeds. Drizzle over the miso dressing.

TOMATO, OLIVE AND WHITE BEAN SALAD

Divide 300g cooked giant couscous or cooked wholemeal pasta between 4 bowls. Add a large handful of rocket to each, then add cannellini or butter beans, grilled artichoke hearts, tomatoes, cucumber and sliced red onions soaked in salted water for 30 minutes. Make a dressing by blitzing together 2 medium tomatoes, 2 tsp vegan balsamic vinegar, 1 garlic clove and a handful of basil. Add olives and capers to the salad, drizzle over the dressing and add some lightly toasted pumpkin seeds or almonds. Garnish with finely torn oregano, thyme or parsley leaves.

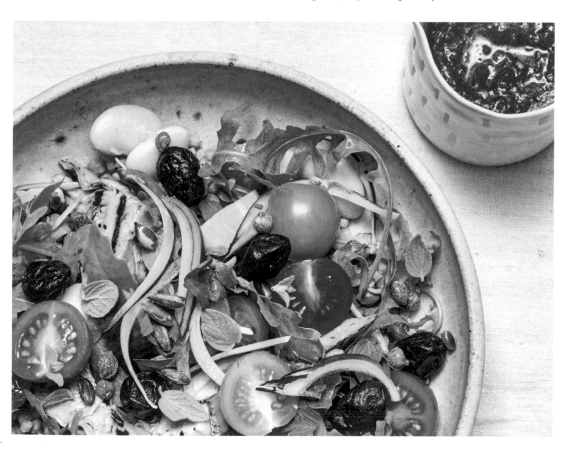

MEDITERRANEAN ROAST VEGETABLE TRAYBAKE

Makes 4–6 portions

2 red onions, cut into thin wedges

2 peppers, any colour, cut into strips

2 courgettes, sliced

1 orange, topped and tailed, then halved and sliced fairly thinly

1 tbsp olive oil (optional)

1 tbsp balsamic or sherry vinegar (optional)

A few sprigs of rosemary and thyme (or dried herbs)

Cloves from ½ a head of garlic, left whole

2 x 400g tin white beans, e.g. cannellini

100ml white wine or stock

50g black olives, pitted

150g cherry tomatoes or larger tomatoes, halved

150g spinach, well washed

To serve

A few basil leaves

Enjoy this easy traybake for a delicious family dinner option – only one pan required. This is a great option to pop in the oven for a midweek feast. If you have younger kids who are not keen on the sight of all those delicious veggies on their plate, you can enjoy any leftovers for a salad topping the next day, or even blitz the cooked ingredients and use them to make a tomato-based sauce to give them with some pasta tomorrow. Sneaky but they'll love it I promise!

Preheat your oven to 200°C/400°F/gas mark 6. Put the onions, peppers, courgettes and orange in a bowl. If using the olive oil, drizzle it over the contents of the bowl. If not, just drizzle over the vinegar – you can drizzle both the oil and the vinegar. Arrange over the base of a large roasting tin. If not using the oil, drizzle 2 tbsp water over the vegetables.

Add the thyme to the roasting tin along with the garlic. Roast for 25 minutes, stirring occasionally. Add the beans and wine or stock to the roasting tin and stir well. Return to the oven for a further 10 minutes.

Add the olives and cherry tomatoes to the roasting tin and cook for a further 10 minutes. At this point the tomatoes should have puffed up and be ready to burst and everything should be lightly browned.

Remove the tin from the oven and stir through the spinach – it will wilt down in the heat almost immediately. Add some torn basil leaves and serve straight away.

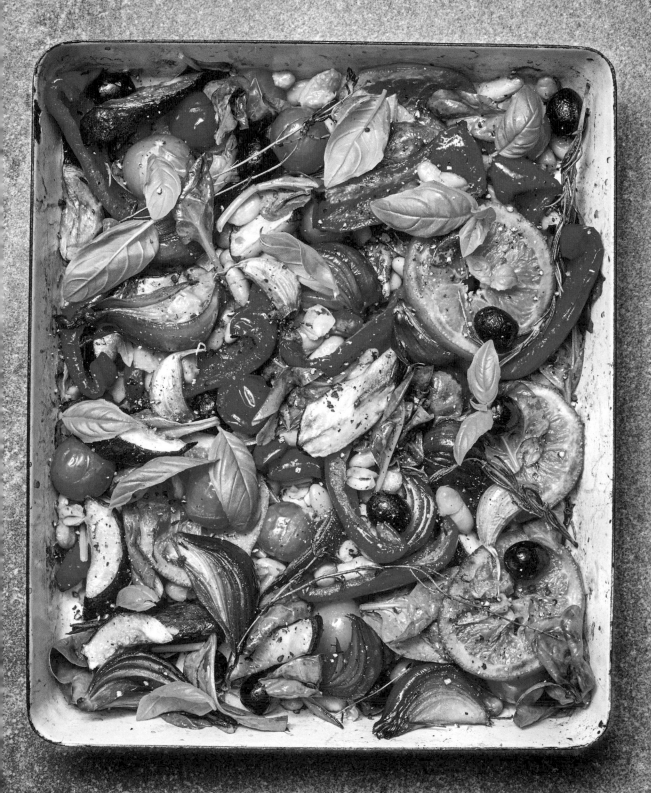

NUT AND VEGGIE ROAST

Makes 4–6 portions

1 tbsp olive oil or a few tbsp water or vegetable stock

1 onion, finely chopped

200g mushrooms, any sort, finely chopped

250g root vegetables, e.g. parsnips, carrots, Jerusalem artichokes, celeriac, grated

2 garlic cloves, crushed

1 tsp dried sage

1 tsp dried thyme

150g cooked brown lentils

100g nuts, roughly chopped – hazelnuts and pecans are especially good

100g cooked chestnuts, crumbled

25g wholemeal breadcrumbs or couscous

3 flax eggs (3 tbsp ground flax seed mixed with 6 tbsp just-boiled water)

50g prunes, roughly chopped (optional)

50ml marsala (optional)

300g spinach, chard, or any kind of kale

Salt and pepper

For the gravy

1 tbsp olive oil or a few tbsp mushroom stock

1 shallot, finely chopped

250g mushrooms, finely chopped

1 garlic clove, finely chopped

A sprig of thyme

50ml marsala or white wine

400ml mushroom stock

2 tsp cornflour or arrowroot

Sunday lunches and Christmas meals call for something special and my nut and veggie roast is super satisfying, If you are cutting out oil, you can use water or stock to fry the ingredients and it's simple to make this switch. Always use a non-stick pan and only add a small amount of water or stock at a time (one or two tablespoons) for the best results.

Preheat your oven to 200°C/400°F/gas mark 6 and line a 900g loaf tin with baking parchment.

If using the oil, heat it in a large frying pan. Alternatively, heat 2 tbsp of water or vegetable stock. Add the onion and mushrooms and cook over a medium heat until the onions have started to soften and the mushrooms have given out their liquid and it has evaporated off. They should be lightly golden in colour around the edges. If not using the oil, you may need to add more stock towards the beginning of the cooking process.

Add the root vegetables and garlic and continue to cook, adding a little more stock if necessary, until they have collapsed down and reduced in volume. Stir in the herbs and remove from the heat.

Put the lentils, nuts, chestnuts and breadcrumbs into a bowl and add the flax eggs. Season with plenty of salt and pepper and add the cooked vegetables. If using, put the prunes in a small saucepan, cover with the marsala and simmer until the liquid has all absorbed. Leave to cool. Cook the spinach, chard or kale in a little water until completely wilted down and squeeze out any excess liquid. Stir through the mixture along with the prunes, if using.

Spoon the mixture into your prepared loaf tin and smooth over the top with a palette knife. Cover with more baking parchment to prevent the loaf from drying out. Bake in the preheated oven for around 1 hour until well browned and piping hot all the way through.

Meanwhile, make the gravy. Heat the oil or 1 tbsp stock in a saucepan and add the shallot. Cook, adding more stock if necessary, until it has softened and caramelised. Add the mushrooms and continue to cook, adding more stock where necessary, until they

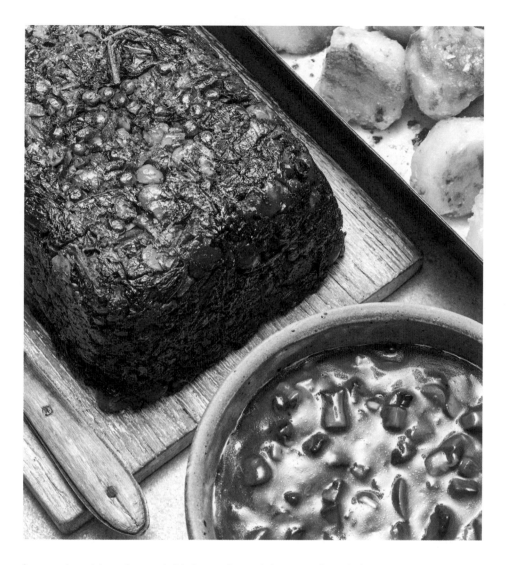

have reduced in volume. Add the garlic and thyme and cook for a couple of minutes. Add the marsala or wine and bring to the boil. Allow to bubble up and reduce to almost nothing, then add the 400ml stock. Cover and simmer for around 10 minutes. If you want a thicker consistency, mix the cornflour or arrowroot with a little water and stir into the gravy. Continue to cook over a medium heat until the gravy thickens.

Serve the nut and veggie roast with the gravy and a wide variety of vegetables.

DESSERTS

Many people think that it is hard to create impressive WFPB desserts without dairy and eggs but this is not true. If you have a sweet tooth, or are looking for a satisfying treat after your main meal, my desserts are easy to make and do not include ingredients that are hard to track down.

PEANUT BUTTER ICE CREAM

Makes 4–6 portions

500ml almond milk

150g unsalted peanut butter

100g almond butter

150g pitted dates

2 tbsp maple or date syrup

2 tsp vanilla extract

A pinch of salt

To serve (optional)

100g vegan chocolate, melted

This shortcut approach to ice cream has a rich and creamy flavour, only contains a few ingredients and is simple to make.

Simply put all the ingredients in a blender and blitz until completely smooth. Pour the mixture into a wide, shallow container. Freeze for 30 minutes, then whisk thoroughly, making sure anything frozen around the edges is well combined with the more liquid centre and that you get plenty of air into the mixture. Refreeze and continue to whisk every 30 minutes–1 hour, each time working in from the edges to the middle, until it is too firm. Continue to freeze until it is solid.

Drizzle with the melted chocolate to serve.

RASPBERRY JELLY

Makes 4–6 portions

350g fresh or frozen raspberries

Up to 300ml apple or grape juice

2 tsp agar-agar powder

Make one of these wobbly jellies bursting with fruity flavours for dessert – they are not just for kids! You can use a bought, pressed fruit juice for this, or coconut water (you may want to add a little sweetener of some sort). It will work with any berry.

Put the raspberries in a heatproof bowl and cover with clingfilm. Set over a saucepan of simmering water and leave for around 30 minutes – the juice will bleed out of the fruit and the fruit will collapse. Line a sieve with muslin and strain the juice. Try to avoid pushing it through as that will result in a cloudy jelly.

Measure the raspberry juice. Separately measure enough apple or grape juice to make the total up to 500ml. Put this juice in a saucepan and sprinkle over the agar-agar powder. Bring to the boil, whisking to help the agar-agar dissolve – it should dissolve within 5 minutes. Remove from the heat and stir in the raspberry juice.

Pour into a 500ml-mould or into individual serving glasses. Do not oil the mould if you are turning the jelly out. You can leave this to set at room temperature or in the fridge but the jelly is best chilled.

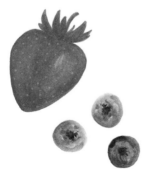

CHOCOLATE MOUSSE

Makes 6 portions

150ml aquafaba

25g caster sugar

150g vegan chocolate

1 tbsp cocoa

50ml almond milk

1 tsp vanilla extract

Salt

Who doesn't love chocolate mousse? This rich and creamy option uses aquafaba, the liquid drained from a can of chickpeas. This makes the mousse light and fluffy, so the perfect dessert for a dinner party or special occasion.

First whisk the aquafaba. This is best done in a stand mixer as it takes time – around 15 minutes – or you could do it with a hand-held electric whisk if you are patient. Start whisking the aquafaba and after a minute or two start adding the sugar, a teaspoon at a time, until it is all completely incorporated. Keep whisking until stiff peaks form.

Meanwhile, put the chocolate in a bowl and set over a saucepan of simmering water until it has melted. Remove from the heat, leave to cool for 5 minutes, then whisk in the cocoa, almond milk and the vanilla extract. Add a pinch of salt. It should be smooth and glossy – if it isn't, add a little more milk and whisk again.

When the chocolate mixture is cool, start folding in the aquafaba. Add a couple of spoons to start with, then add the rest. Fold with a spatula or large metal spoon, trying to make sure you keep as much air in as possible, until it is completely combined. Spoon into 6 large ramekins and put in the fridge to chill and set. Serve with a little extra chocolate grated over it.

NB – the cocoa content of the chocolate is up to you. If this is for children, you might choose one with a lower cocoa content; if this is for a dinner party, a higher cocoa content might be preferable. Any vegan chocolate will work.

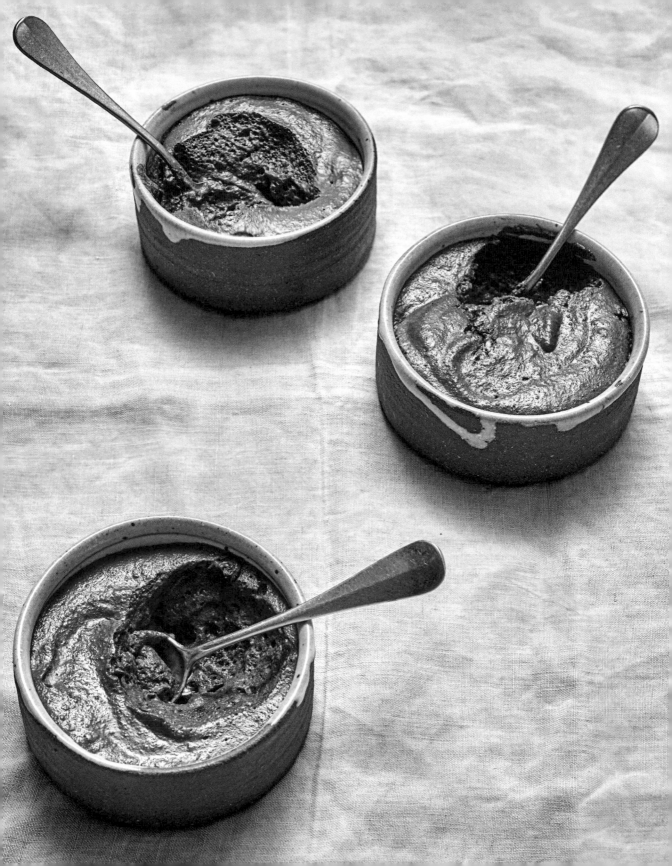

BANANA BREAD

Makes 12 generous slices

125g wholemeal plain flour
(spelt also a good option)

1 tsp baking powder

½ tsp bicarbonate of soda

100g light soft brown sugar or
coconut sugar or maple syrup

2 large bananas

80g nut butter or tahini

1 tsp cider vinegar

125ml soy milk

1 tsp vanilla extract

60ml just-boiled water

2 tbsp ground flax seed

100g raisins or sultanas,
soaked in 100ml strong tea

Salt

Use your ripe bananas to make my version of banana bread, which is a great treat to enjoy with your cuppa. For a comforting dessert, this also tastes great with a little custard (vegan custard can be shop-bought nowadays or you can make your own using my recipe on page 254).

Preheat the oven to 180°C/350°F/gas mark 4, and either line a 900g loaf tin with baking parchment or brush with cake release.

Mix together the flour, baking powder, bicarbonate of soda and sugar. Add a generous pinch of salt and set aside.

Mash the bananas into a bowl and add the nut butter or tahini, continuing to mash together until well combined. Add the cider vinegar to the milk and let it stand for a few minutes until it thickens. Stir in the vanilla extract. Add the just boiled water to the flax meal and let it stand for 5 minutes. Add the thickened milk and flax meal to the bananas and combine.

Add the wet ingredients to the dry and mix until just combined – you need to try to keep the stirring to a minimum. Drain the raisins and stir these in too. Pour into the prepared tin and bake for around 1 hour until well risen, well browned and firm on top. Leave in the tin to cool then transfer to an airtight tin for up to a week.

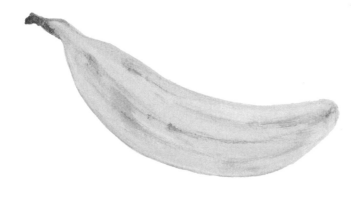

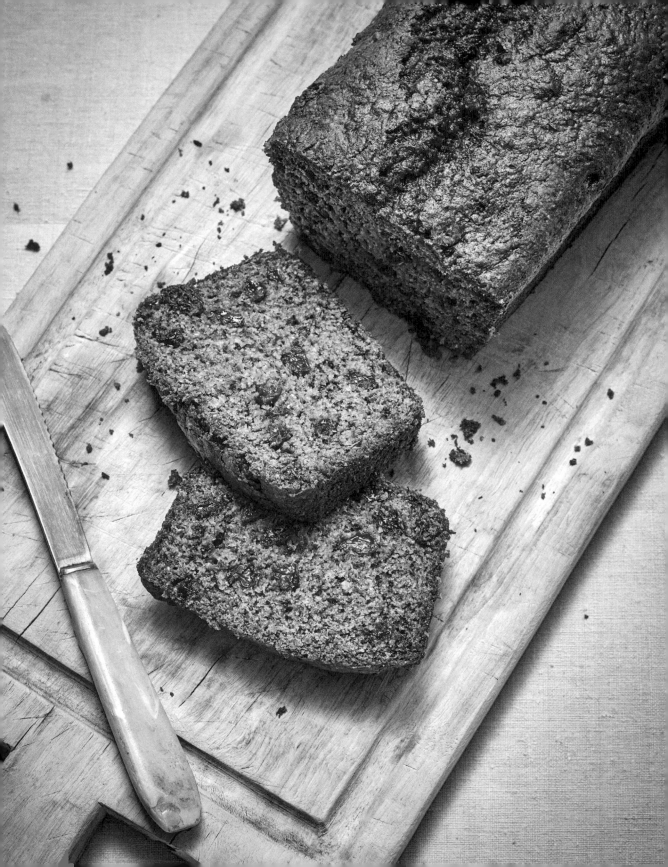

FRUIT COBBLER

Makes 4–6 portions

For the base

3 peaches, cut into wedges

100g blueberries

1 tbsp coconut sugar or soft light brown sugar

1 tsp cornflour

½ tsp ground cinnamon

For the topping

100g wholemeal self-raising flour

75g ground almonds

1 tbsp baking powder

2 tbsp coconut or soft light brown sugar

150ml plant-based milk (almond is good here)

A few drops of almond or vanilla extract

1 tsp cider vinegar

1 flax egg (1 tbsp ground flax seed mixed with 2 tbsp just-boiled water)

For the custard

500ml plant-based milk

2 tbsp light soft brown sugar or maple syrup

1 tsp vanilla extract

3 tbsp cornflour

This warming recipe is a classic comfort food. I've made this with fresh peaches and blueberries, but it can also be made with apples, pears, plums or any frozen packets of mixed fruits, such as fruits of the forest.

Bird's custard powder is vegan and oil free if you get the original powder, not the instant variety. It can be made with plant-based milk – the only real difference between using this and the cornflour recipe I give here is annatto powder, which gives it the colour.

Preheat the oven to 180°C/350°F/gas mark 4. Arrange the fruit in the base of an ovenproof dish. Mix the sugar, cornflour and cinnamon together and sprinkle over the fruit. Stir to combine.

If using apples, mix them with the base ingredients and add them to a large saucepan over a medium heat to soften with a dash of water or apple juice for 5 minutes before stirring in any berries you might want.

To make the topping, put the flour in a bowl with the ground almonds, baking powder and sugar. Mix the plant-based milk with the almond or vanilla extract and cider vinegar, then stir in the flax egg. Pour the wet ingredients into the dry and combine, keeping the mixing to a minimum. Drop heaped tablespoons of the mixture over the fruit.

Bake in the oven for 30–35 minutes until the topping is brown and the juice from the fruit is bubbling through.

To make the custard, put 400ml of the plant-based milk in a saucepan and the rest in a large bowl or jug. Heat the 400ml milk with the sugar and vanilla extract, stirring until the sugar has completely dissolved. Mix the remaining milk with the cornflour.

Just before the milk boils, pour it into the jug, stirring constantly, then pour everything back into the saucepan. Heat, gradually bringing to the boil, stirring constantly, until the custard thickens. It may suddenly start thickening very quickly on the base of the saucepan – if so, stir or whisk furiously to make sure you don't get any lumps. Transfer to a jug and serve with the fruit cobbler.

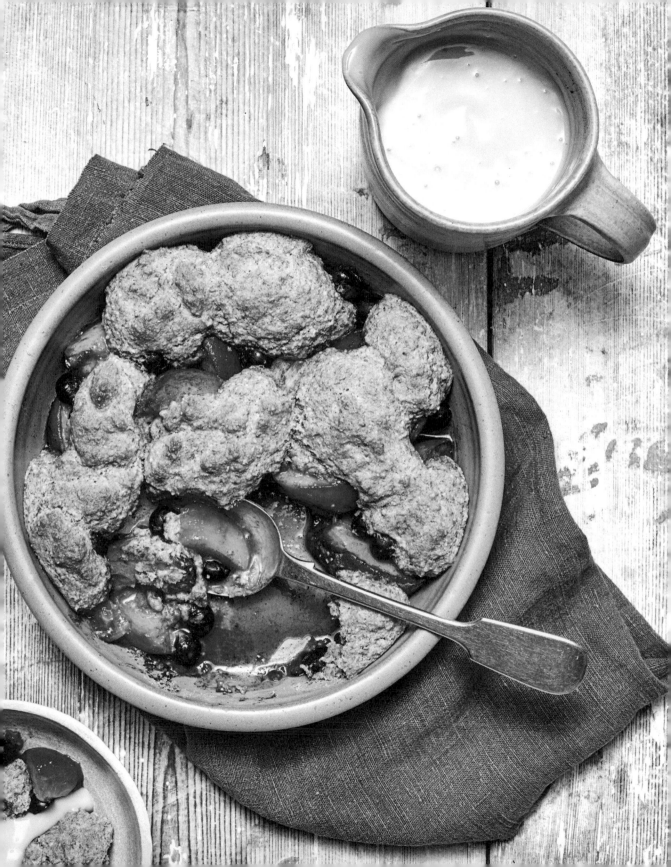

RICE PUDDING WITH FRUIT COMPOTE

Makes 4–6 portions

3–4 cardamom pods

1 cinnamon stick

1 piece pared lime zest

150g rice – you can use pretty much any sort, but short grain is best

1.2 litres almond milk

50g light brown sugar or coconut sugar or date syrup

A pinch of salt

Nutmeg, for grating

For the compote

500g frozen or fresh berries, cherries, pears, plums or apricots, roughly chopped

½ tsp ground cinnamon

½ tsp ground ginger

2 tbsp light brown sugar or coconut sugar or date syrup

2 tsp cornflour (optional)

Salt

This lightly spiced and creamy pudding can be eaten hot or cold and is good with any very ripe fruit – try slices of mango or peaches, or a compote with orchard fruit or berries when fresh fruit is not available.

I've tried making this with a few different plant-based milks and have found that almond milk works best. If you want to use coconut milk, use the coconut milk drink in a carton, rather than the tinned version as this has a lot of oil and will separate as you cook.

Toast the cardamom and cinnamon stick in a saucepan until they are giving out a strong aroma. Add the lime zest and rice and continue to toast for a further minute. Pour in the almond milk and whichever type of sweetener you are using along with the pinch of salt. Slowly bring to the boil, then reduce the heat right down and partially cover. Cook, stirring regularly to prevent it catching, until the rice has cooked through and the liquid has thickened – this can take up to 1 hour. Once cooked, remove the cardamom pods and cinnamon stick.

Grate a little nutmeg over the cooked rice pudding and serve with the fruit compote.

FRUIT COMPOTE

Put the fruit into a saucepan. If you are using frozen fruit, simply add the spices, a pinch of salt and your choice of sweetener. If you are using fresh fruit, add 50ml water to help the fruit get started. Simmer gently until the fruit has softened and started to break down. If doing so produces a lot of liquid, you may want to thicken it slightly. If so, mix the cornflour with a little cold water and stir into the fruit. Continue to cook, stirring constantly, until the sauce thickens. Remove from the heat. This will keep in the fridge for up to a week and can also be frozen.

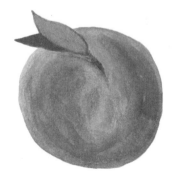

SNACKS

If you are looking for quick and satisfying treats, so you are not hunting around in your cupboards for crisps and other convenience snacks, these recipes will satisfy your hunger and are all WFPB. They include sweet and savoury options that will keep kids happy too!

TRAIL MIX

This makes a generous 450g tub

100g almonds (preferably skin on for fibre)

100g cashew nuts

50g pumpkin seeds

25g unsweetened coconut flakes

50g unsweetened dried mango, diced if in strips

50g banana chips, crumbled (see recipe if you need oil free)

50g raisins or sultanas or chopped dates

15g dried or crystallised ginger, finely chopped

¼ tsp ground cinnamon

¼ tsp ground cardamom

¼ tsp ground turmeric

I've found trail mix brilliant for adding my kids' favourite nuts and fruits together. My boys have so much fun choosing ingredients to add together and mix. I've introduced a few warm spices and crystallised ginger for a tropical taste. Look for dried fruit that is not coated in sugar and oil as this will be a healthier choice.

Simply mix all the ingredients together. If you find it difficult to find dried fruit which has not been coated in oil (this is common, it stops fruit from clumping together), rinse the fruit in boiling water, then drain and arrange on kitchen towel until completely dry.

If you want to include dried bananas, those commercially available are usually fried in coconut oil. They are easy to make at home without adding oil or sugar. Simply slice bananas quite thinly and toss in lemon or lime juice to prevent browning. Arrange on baking parchment over a baking tray. Set your oven to its lowest temperature and leave the bananas in the oven with the door slightly ajar for several hours (start checking after 3 hours) until they are crisp and dehydrated. Alternatively, use a dehydrator if you have one. Store in an airtight container.

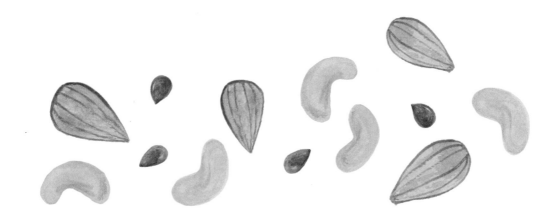

POPCORN

Makes enough for 4 to snack

1 tsp walnut oil (optional)

100g popping corn kernels

Savoury

½ tsp salt

½ tsp smoked chilli powder (optional)

Sweet

½ tsp ground cinnamon

A little maple or date syrup (optional)

Popcorn is always a hit and this simple recipe is very easy. You can use oil for popping (walnut, olive, or avocado) but if you are cutting out oil it can also be dry popped.

Heat the oil in a large saucepan if using – keep the temperature at medium. If not using the oil, just heat your saucepan over a medium heat for a few minutes.

Add the popcorn and put a lid on. Leave covered, shaking every so often until you hear the corn start popping. It's really important that if you aren't using the oil, you shake the pan very frequently – if you don't, the underside of the popcorn may burn before it is hot enough to start popping.

The popping noise will start slowly and gradually speed up and die down again. When you've gone for at least 30 seconds without hearing a pop, remove the popcorn from the heat. Transfer to a bowl.

To flavour, sprinkle with your choice of sweet or savoury coatings.

BANANA AND CHOCOLATE CATERPILLAR

Makes 2 portions

2 bananas, sliced

juice of ½ lime

2 tbsp nut butter – cashew or almond probably works best

1 tbsp date syrup

2 tsp cocoa or cacao powder

A pinch of ground cinnamon (optional)

2 tsp white sesame seeds

A few grapes

A few currants

Salt

This is a great way to introduce WFPB snacks for children who will love helping you prepare this delicious treat. Even the fussiest eaters will enjoy this!

Toss the bananas in the lime juice and set aside.

Make the chocolate paste by mixing together the nut butter, date syrup, cocoa or cacao powder and cinnamon. Add a pinch of salt. You should have a thick, malleable paste.

Sandwich the paste with the bananas into two wiggly lines, finishing with a round of banana facing up. Sprinkle the sesame seeds over the chocolate for a dappled effect. Cut the grapes in half and then into slices and arrange on either side of the banana caterpillars for legs. Press currants into the upturned round of banana for eyes and draw a smile on with a skewer. Use grape stems for antennae.

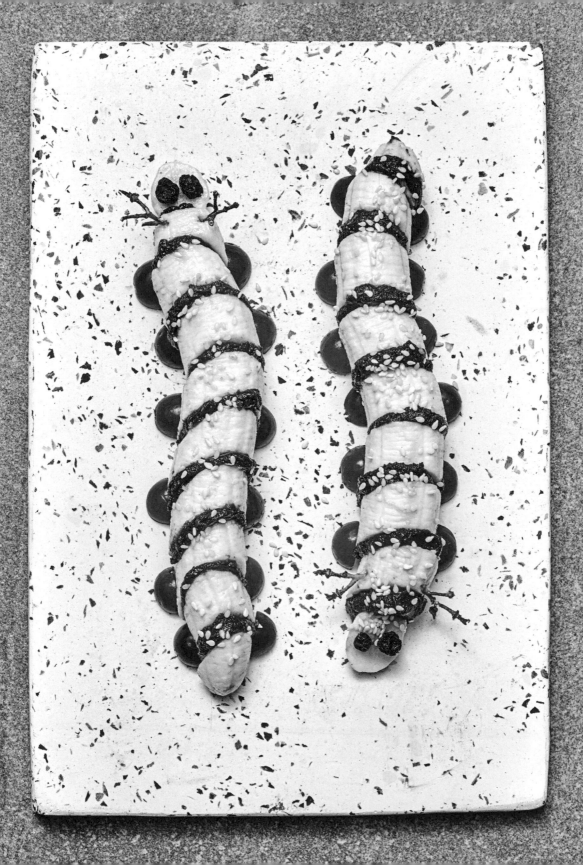

OIL-FREE HUMMUS WITH CRUDITÉS

Makes enough for 4 people to snack on

1 x 400g can chickpeas

Juice of 1 lemon

2 tbsp tahini

1 garlic clove, finely chopped

Salt

To top

A sprinkling of za'atar or other herbs

Sesame seeds

Pomegranate seeds

To serve

Batons of carrots, cucumber and peppers, cauliflower florets, cherry tomatoes – anything you like!

Hummus is a favourite with plant-based eaters. This recipe can be made with virtually any type of bean instead of the chickpeas.

Put all the ingredients into a food processor, reserving some of the chickpea liquid, and blend until smooth. Add some chickpea liquid or water if the hummus seems too thick. Taste and season with salt. Alternatively, you can mash the chickpeas with a potato masher.

WHITE BEAN, ARTICHOKE AND LEMON

Makes 4 portions

1 x 400g tin white beans

1 x tin artichoke hearts in water

Zest and juice of 1 lemon

1 garlic clove, crushed

2 tbsp plant-based milk

Salt and pepper

This dip is another way to enjoy plants and can also be enjoyed with crudités. I use jars of artichokes in water or brine, as opposed to the ones in oil.

Simply put all the ingredients into a food processor and season with salt and pepper. Pulse until you have a thick, coarse purée.

GUACAMOLE, SALSA AND VEGAN CHEESE DIP WITH NACHOS

Makes 4–6 portions

If you are looking for treats to enjoy while watching a film or when you have friends over, nachos are always a big hit. Here are three different dips to enjoy with yours. For the vegan cheese and onion dip, I find the best way to soften the cashews is to soak them overnight in filtered water, so they are easier to break down into a smooth paste.

For the guacamole

Zest and juice of 1 lime

½ tsp ground cumin

¼ red onion, very finely chopped

2 avocados

A few sprigs of coriander, finely chopped

Salt

For the vegan cheese and onion dip

100g cashew nuts

50ml plant-based milk

1 tsp garlic powder

1 tsp onion granules

2 tbsp nutritional yeast

½ small onion, very finely chopped

1 tsp white wine vinegar

Salt

GUACAMOLE

Squeeze the lime juice into a bowl and add the zest, cumin, red onion and ½ tsp salt. Peel and dice the avocados and mash lightly. Add to the lime juice mixture, then stir in the coriander. Taste for seasoning and adjust if necessary.

VEGAN CHEESE AND ONION DIP

Put the cashew nuts in a saucepan and cover with water. Bring to the boil and simmer for 15 minutes until soft. Strain and put into a blender with the plant-based milk, garlic powder, onion granules and nutritional yeast. Blend until smooth – this may take several minutes. If you feel your blender is not up to the job, when everything is broken down you can finish it off by pushing through a fine sieve. Season with salt and stir in the onion and white wine vinegar. Chill for at least an hour before serving. It will keep in the fridge stored in an airtight container for a few days.

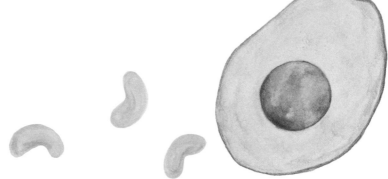
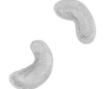

For the tomato salsa

4 tomatoes, stem removed, and the seeds and flesh finely chopped

½ red onion, finely chopped

Juice of ½ lime

2 tsp sherry or red wine vinegar

A pinch of smoked chilli powder (optional)

A few sprigs coriander, finely chopped

Salt and pepper

For the nachos

1 pack tortillas (preferably small corn ones), cut into triangles

Juice of 1 lime

Smoked chilli powder (optional)

Dried oregano (optional)

Salt

TOMATO SALSA

Simply mix all the ingredients together and season with plenty of salt and pepper. Leave to stand at room temperature to allow the flavours to meld.

NACHOS

Preheat the oven to 170°C/325°F/gas mark 3. Arrange the tortillas over a couple of baking trays. Combine the lime juice with 1 tbsp water and sprinkle over the tortillas. Sprinkle with salt and the smoked chilli powder and/or the oregano if you like. Bake in the oven for around 15 minutes until crisp and curled up. Make sure they seem completely dried out – if not, leave for a little longer. Remove from the oven and leave to cool before enjoying alongside your dips.

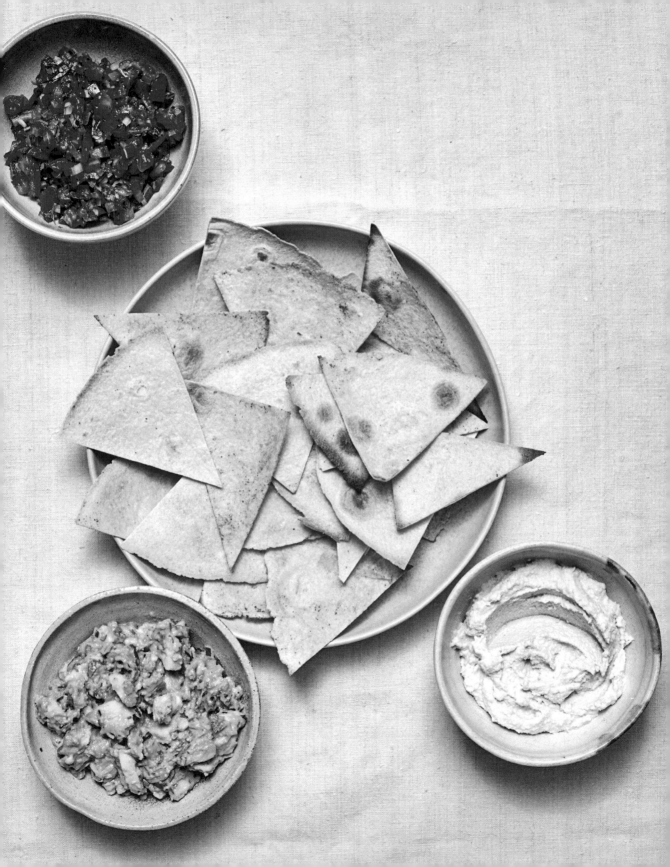

CONCLUSION

'When we try to pick out anything by itself, we find it hitched to everything else in the Universe.'

John Muir

I hope you now agree that there is no doubt that nutrition plays a huge and central role in our health, and therefore in our happiness. Changing what is on our plate creates momentum to help us form other healthy habits too, and ultimately helps us to build a body and brain from optimal ingredients. But vitality is about so much more than this. I have met some patients with extremely well planned out diets who struggle with anxiety. I have met others who exercise daily and yet burn out from lack of sleep. Our thoughts and emotions – ruminating on the past or worrying about the future – can also drive our habits and choices because they are ultimately in charge of what we do, think and feel.

This book has been a roadmap for you to harness the power of nutrition. My hope is that the evidence presented and the practical tips and recipes you can try will give you a head start in beginning to understand how powerful your body and mind can truly be.

You have all you need within you. I feel confident that this way of living will bring you a greater understanding of this universal truth, and be a part of your own path to health and happiness.

Now more than ever, we need new ways to look at the world.

The coronavirus pandemic of 2020 gave all of us a real sense that the old ways of living were not working.

Could this unique situation in history have been predicted? Viral epidemics have been increasing in frequency over the last few decades. Think back to other recent challenges we have faced and you will quickly see a pattern. Spanish flu came from poultry, swine flu came from pigs and avian flu came from birds. We've also seen SARS-CoV (from civets), MERS-CoV (from camels) and of course now SARS-CoV-2, which was likely to have come about from the destruction of bat habitats and human use of animals in wet markets. Whatever the origins of this virus, we know that diseases that spread from the use of animals (zoonotic diseases) infect 2.5 billion people every year.

Intensive farming methods have also been connected to illness. We have already touched on the impact that antibiotics in the food chain have on our health. Intensive animal farming is also the cause of salmonella (a serious outbreak in the UK happened in 1988 and infections are rising again) and E. coli infections.

How can you ensure you are as strong and healthy as you can be to take on future pandemics?

Do you need to eat meat, fish and dairy every day, if at all?

What can you do to change your lifestyle to make you and your family better equipped to deal with whatever disease life might throw at you?

My hope is that you will embrace the suggestions in this book as a way to live that will give you the tools you need for a happier, healthier life, as well as a more sustainable world.

Alongside caring for our personal health, I want to touch again on the planet and global health – now and in the future. The science on climate change is now clear – unless we take action there will be catastrophic consequences. An inhospitable world for all of us. Air pollution, increased temperatures, reduced water supplies and disrupted food supplies can and will affect everyone in the future – unless we do something today.

As Brené Brown said, the pandemic and unrest of 2020 was 'a massive experiment in collective vulnerability'. Let's be vulnerable and brave. Let's try new things to improve our health and make a better future for our children and grandchildren and those who come after them too.

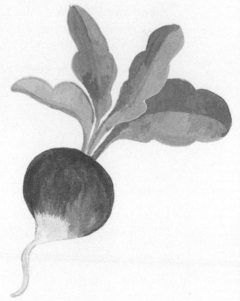

Share a delicious wholefoods plant-based meal with your friends. Do something kind to make someone feel good. Introduce the people you love to a new way of thinking. The Plant Power way.

Much love,
Dr Gemma Newman

KEY REFERENCES

Eating more plants is healing. But I don't want you to just take my word for it. Within this book I have compiled nearly 600 references from journal articles spanning many decades and from many sources. It was really important to me to be able to share compelling evidence, so you could feel reassured that the changes you make are both evidence based and steeped in science. There were in fact so many references, that we were unable to include them all in print. All references are available to view on my website, www.gemmanewman.com. They are grouped by chapter to make it as easy as possible for you to find the studies that are of interest to you.

Below is an abridged version of a few selected studies that I thought may be of most interest; but please do head to my website for a full and detailed summary of the evidence presented.

INTRODUCTION

Barnard ND, Goldman DM, Loomis JF, *et al.*, 'Plant-Based Diets for Cardiovascular Safety and Performance in Endurance Sports', *Nutrients* (2019); 11(1): 130. doi: 10.3390/nu11010130.

Trapp D., Knez W., Sinclair W, 'Could a vegetarian diet reduce exercise-induced oxidative stress? A review of the literature', *Journal of Sports Sciences* (2010); 28: 1261–8.

Sutliffe JT, Wilson LD, de Heer HD, Foster RL, Carnot MJ, 'C-reactive protein response to a vegan lifestyle intervention', *Complementary Therapies in Medicine* (2015); 23(1): 32–7.

Kim H, Caulfield LE, Garcia-Larsen V, Steffen LM, Coresh J, Rebholz CM, 'Plant-Based Diets Are Associated With a Lower Risk of Incident Cardiovascular Disease, Cardiovascular Disease Mortality, and All-Cause Mortality in a General Population of Middle-Aged Adults', *Journal of the American Heart Association* (2019); 8(16): e012865. doi: 10.1161/JAHA.119.012865

Kim H, Caulfield LE, Rebholz CM, 'Healthy Plant-Based Diets Are Associated with Lower Risk of All-Cause Mortality in US Adults', *Journal of Nutrition* (2018); 148(4): 624–31. doi: 10.1093/jn/nxy019.

Turner-Mcgrievy GM, Wirth MD, Shivappa N, Wingard EE, Fayad R, Wilcox S, *et al.*, 'Randomization to plant-based dietary approaches leads to larger short-term improvements in dietary inflammatory index scores and macronutrient intake compared with diets that contain meat', *Nutrition Research* (2015); 35: 97–106.

Najjar RS, Moore CE, Montgomery BD, 'Consumption of a defined, plant-based diet reduces lipoprotein(a), inflammation, and other atherogenic lipoproteins and particles within 4 weeks', *Clininical Cardiology* (2018); 41: 1062–68.

Kim MK, Cho SW, Park YK, 'Long-term vegetarians have low oxidative stress, body fat, and cholesterol levels', *Nutrition Research and Practice* (2012); 6: 155–61.

Alexander S, Ostfeld RJ, Allen K, Williams KA, 'A plant-based diet and hypertension', *Journal of Geriatric Cardiology* (2017); 14(5): 327–30. doi: 10.11909/j.issn.1671-5411.2017.05.014.

Whelton SP, Hyre AD, Pedersen B, Yi Y, Whelton PK, He J, 'Effect of dietary fiber intake on blood pressure: a meta-analysis of randomized, controlled clinical trials', *Journal of Hypertension* (2005); 23: 475–81.

Rodriguez-Leyva D, Weighell W, Edel AL,

LaVallee R, Dibrov E, Pinneker R, Maddaford TG, Ramjiawan B, Aliani M, Guzman R, *et al.*, 'Potent antihypertensive action of dietary flaxseed in hypertensive patients', *Hypertension* (2013); 62: 1081–9.

Dodin S, Lemay A, Jacques H, Legare F, Forest J-C, Masse B, 'The effects of flaxseed dietary supplement on lipid profile, bone mineral density, and symptoms in menopausal women: a randomized, double-blind, wheat germ placebo-controlled clinical trial', *The Journal of Clinical Endocrinology & Metabolism* (2005); 90: 1390–7.

WHAT IS A WHOLEFOODS PLANT-BASED DIET?

GBD 2017 Diet Collaborators, 'Health effects of dietary risks in 195 countries, 1990–2017: a systematic analysis for the Global Burden of Disease Study 2017', *The Lancet* (2019); 393(10184): 1958–72. doi: 10.1016/S0140-6736(19)30041-8.

Ceballos G, Ehrlich PR, Barnosky AD, García A, Pringle RM, Palmer TM, 'Accelerated modern human-induced species losses: Entering the sixth mass extinction', *Science Advances* (2015); 1(5): e1400253. Published 2015 Jun 19. doi: 10.1126/sciadv.1400253.

Poore J, Nemecek T, 'Reducing food's environmental impacts through producers and consumers. *Science* (2018); 360(6392): 987–92. [published correction appears in *Science* (2019); 363(6429)]

EAT Lancet Commission: https://eatforum.org/eat-lancet-commission/eat-lancet-commission-summary-report/

WHY IS A WFPB DIET HEALTHY?

Rui Hai Liu, 'Health benefits of fruit and vegetables are from additive and synergistic combinations of phytochemicals', *The American Journal of Clinical Nutrition* (2003); 78(3): 517S–520S.

LONGEVITY – WHO LIVES TO 100?

Buettner D, Skemp S, 'Blue Zones: Lessons From the World's Longest Lived', *American Journal of Lifestyle Medicine* (2016); 10(5): 318–21.

Dellara F. Terry, Vikki G. Nolan, Stacy L. Andersen, Thomas T. Perls, Richard Cawthon, 'Association of Longer Telomeres With Better Health in Centenarians', *The Journals of Gerontology* (Series A, 2008); 63(8): 809–12.

Ornish D, Lin J, Chan JM, *et al.* 'Effect of comprehensive lifestyle changes on telomerase activity and telomere length in men with biopsy-proven low-risk prostate cancer: 5-year follow-up of a descriptive pilot study', *The Lancet Oncology* (2013); 14(11): 1112–20.

Sansbury BE, Hill BG, 'Regulation of obesity and insulin resistance by nitric oxide', *Free Radical Biology and Medicine* (2014); 73: 383–99.

Kobayashi J, Ohtake K, Uchida H, 'NO-Rich Diet for Lifestyle-Related Diseases', *Nutrients* (2015); 7(6): 4911–37.

Cornu M, Albert V, Hall MN, 'mTOR in aging, metabolism, and cancer', *Current Opinion in Genetics & Development* (2013); 23(1): 53–62.

Kitada M, Ogura Y, Monno I, Koya D, 'The impact of dietary protein intake on longevity and metabolic health', *EBioMedicine* (2019); 43: 632–40.

EAT MORE AND WEIGH LESS

Wang H, Dwyer-Lindgren L, Lofgren KT, *et al.*, '1970-2010: a systematic analysis for the Global Burden of Disease Study 2010', *The Lancet* (2015); 380(9859).

Mann, T., *Secrets from the Eating Lab: The Science of Weight Loss, the Myth of Willpower and Why You Should Never Diet Again* (Harper Wave 2017).

Newell BR, Shanks DR, 'Unconscious influences on decision making: a critical review', *Behavioral and Brain Sciences* (2014); 37(1): 1–19. doi: 10.1017/S0140525X12003214 as discussed in a lecture by Professor Paul Chadwick, UCL.

Koithan M, Devika J, 'New Approaches to Nutritional Therapy', *The Journal for Nurse Practitioners* (2010); 6(10): 805–6.

Fuhrman J, Sarter B, Glaser D, Acocella S, 'Changing perceptions of hunger on a high nutrient density diet', *Nutrition Journal* (2010); 9: 51.

Karlsen MC, Rogers G, Miki A, *et al.,* 'Theoretical Food and Nutrient Composition of Whole-Food Plant-Based and Vegan Diets Compared to Current Dietary Recommendations', *Nutrients* (2019); 11(3): 625.

Tonstad S, Butler T, Yan R, Fraser GE, 'Type of vegetarian diet, body weight, and prevalence of type 2 diabetes', *Diabetes Care* (2009); 32(5): 791–6.

Siahpush M, Tibbits M, Shaikh RA, Singh GK, Sikora Kessler A, Huang TT, 'Dieting Increases the Likelihood of Subsequent Obesity and BMI Gain: Results from a Prospective Study of an Australian National Sample', *International Journal of Behavioral Medicine* (2015); 22(5): 662–71.

Masterson TD, Brand J, Lowe MR, *et al.,* 'Relationships Among Dietary Cognitive Restraint, Food Preferences, and Reaction Times', *Frontiers in Psychology* (2019); 10: 2256.

Wright N, Wilson L, Smith M, Duncan B, McHugh P, 'The BROAD study: A randomised controlled trial using a whole food plant-based diet in the community for obesity, ischaemic heart disease or diabetes', *Nutrition & Diabetes* (2017); 7(3): e256.

Matheson EM, King DE, Everett CJ, 'Healthy lifestyle habits and mortality in overweight and obese individuals', *The Journal of the American Board of Family Medicine* (2012); 25(1): 9–15.

Klementova M, Thieme L, Haluzik M, *et al.,* 'A Plant-Based Meal Increases Gastrointestinal Hormones and Satiety More Than an Energy- and Macronutrient-Matched Processed-Meat Meal in T2D, Obese, and Healthy Men: A Three-Group Randomized Crossover Study', *Nutrients* (2019); 11(1): 157.

Li H, Li J, Shen Y, Wang J, Zhou D, 'Legume Consumption and All-Cause and Cardiovascular Disease Mortality', *BioMed Research International* (2017); 2017: 8450618.

Higgins JA, 'Whole grains, legumes, and the subsequent meal effect: implications for blood glucose control and the role of fermentation', *Journal of Nutrition and Metaboilsm* (2012); 2012: 829238.

McRae MP, 'Health Benefits of Dietary Whole Grains: An Umbrella Review of Meta-analyses', *Journal of Chiropractic Medicine* (2017); 16(1): 10–18.

HEART HEALTH

Benson TW, Weintraub NL, Kim HW, *et al.,* 'A single high-fat meal provokes pathological erythrocyte remodeling and increases myeloperoxidase levels: implications for acute coronary syndrome', *Laboratory Investigation* (2018); 98(10): 1300–10.

Hooper L, Martin N, Jimoh OF, Kirk C, Foster E, Abdelhamid AS, 'Reduction in saturated fat intake for cardiovascular disease', *The Cochrane Database of Systematic Reviews* (2020); 5: CD011737.

Ginsberg HN, Karmally W, Siddiqui M, *et al.,* 'A dose-response study of the effects of dietary cholesterol on fasting and postprandial lipid and lipoprotein metabolism in healthy young men', *Arteriosclerosis, Thrombosis, and Vascular Biology* (1994); 14(4): 576–86.

Fred H. Mattson, R. A. Volpenhein, B. A. Erickson, 'Effect of Plant Sterol Esters on the Absorption of Dietary Cholesterol', *The Journal of Nutrition* (1977); 107(7): 1139–46.

Hiroshi Hara, Satoko Haga, Yoritaka Aoyama, Shuhachi Kiriyama, 'Short-Chain Fatty Acids Suppress Cholesterol Synthesis in Rat Liver and Intestine', *The Journal of Nutrition* (1999); 129(5): 942–48.

Houston MC, 'The importance of potassium in managing hypertension', *Current Hypertension Reports* (2011); 13(4): 309–17.

Zhang X, Li Y, Del Gobbo LC, *et al.,* 'Effects of Magnesium Supplementation on Blood Pressure: A Meta-Analysis of Randomized Double-Blind Placebo-Controlled Trials', *Hypertension* (2016); 68(2): 324–33.

Alferink, L.J.M., Erler, N.S., de Knegt, R.J. *et al.,* 'Adherence to a plant-based, high-fibre dietary pattern is related to regression of non-alcoholic fatty liver disease in an elderly population', *European Journal of Epidemiology* (2020).

Threapleton DE, Greenwood DC, Evans CE, *et al.,* 'Dietary fibre intake and risk of cardiovascular disease: systematic review and meta-analysis', *BMJ* (2013); 347: f6879.

Kerley CP, 'A Review of Plant-based Diets to Prevent and Treat Heart Failure', *Cardiac Failure Review* (2018); 4(1): 54–61.

de Lorgeril M, Salen P, Martin JL, Monjaud I, Delaye J, Mamelle N, 'Mediterranean diet, traditional risk factors, and the rate of cardiovascular complications after myocardial infarction: final report of the Lyon Diet Heart Study', *Circulation* (1999); 99(6): 779–85.

Ornish D, Brown SE, Scherwitz LW, *et al.,* 'Can lifestyle changes reverse coronary heart disease? The Lifestyle Heart Trial', *The Lancet* (1990); 336(8708): 129–33. doi: 10.1016/0140-6736(90)91656-u.

Esselstyn CB, 'A plant-based diet and coronary artery disease: a mandate for effective therapy', *Journal of Geriatric Cardiology* (2017); 14(5): 317–20.

Arnett DK, Blumenthal RS, Albert MA, *et al.,* '2019 ACC/AHA Guideline on the Primary Prevention of Cardiovascular Disease: A Report of the American College of Cardiology/American Heart Association Task Force on Clinical Practice Guidelines'.

Boden WE, O'Rourke RA, Teo KK, *et al.* 'Optimal medical therapy with or without PCI for stable coronary disease', *The New England Journal of Medicine* (2007); 356(15): 1503–16.

Ounpuu S, Negassa A, Yusuf S, 'INTER-HEART: A global study of risk factors for acute myocardial infarction', *American Heart Journal* (2001); 141(5): 711–21.

HOW FAT INFLUENCES OUR HEALTH

Mustad VA, Etherton TD, Cooper AD, *et al.,* 'Reducing saturated fat intake is associated with increased levels of LDL receptors on mononuclear cells in healthy men and women', *Journal of Lipid Research* (1997); 38(3): 459–68.

Ginter E, Simko V, 'New data on harmful effects of trans-fatty acids', *Bratislava Medical Journal* (2016); 117(5): 251–53.

Hayes J, Benson G, 'What the Latest Evidence Tells Us About Fat and Cardiovascular Health', *Diabetes Spectrum* (2016); 29(3): 171–75. doi: 10.2337/diaspect.29.3.171.

Dórea JG, 'Persistent, bioaccumulative

and toxic substances in fish: human health considerations', *Science of the Total Environment* (2008); 400(1–3): 93–114. doi: 10.1016/j.scitotenv.2008.06.017.

Laffoley, D.Baxter, J. M, 'IUCN Report Explaining ocean warming: causes, scale, effects and consequences', (2016): 456.

Tuso P, Stoll SR, Li WW, 'A plant-based diet, atherogenesis, and coronary artery disease prevention', *The Permanente Journal* (2015); 19(1): 62–7. doi: 10.7812/TPP/14-036.

RETHINKING CANCER

Donaldson MS, 'Nutrition and cancer: a review of the evidence for an anti-cancer diet', *Nutrition Journal* (2004); 3: 19.

Contaldo F, Santarpia L, Cioffi I, Pasanisi F, 'Nutrition Transition and Cancer', *Nutrients* (2020); 12(3): 795.

Seitz HK, Becker P, 'Alcohol metabolism and cancer risk', *Alcohol Research & Health* (2007); 30(1): 38–47.

Zheng W, Lee SA, 'Well-done meat intake, heterocyclic amine exposure, and cancer risk', *Nutrition and Cancer* (2009); 61(4): 437–46.

Skog KI, Johansson MA, Jägerstad MI, 'Carcinogenic heterocyclic amines in model systems and cooked foods: a review on formation, occurrence and intake', *Food and Chemical Toxicology* (1998); 36(9–10): 879–96.

Platt KL, Edenharder R, Aderhold S, Muckel E, Glatt H, 'Fruits and vegetables protect against the genotoxicity of heterocyclic aromatic amines activated by human xenobiotic-metabolizing enzymes expressed in immortal mammalian cells', *Mutation Research* (2010); 703(2): 90–8.

Cross AJ, Peters U, Kirsh VA, *et al.*, 'A prospective study of meat and meat mutagens and prostate cancer risk', *Cancer Research* (2005); 65(24): 11779–84.

Sabine Rohrmann, Sea-Uck Lukas Jung, Jakob Linseisen, Wolfgang Pfau, 'Dietary intake of meat and meat-derived heterocyclic aromatic amines and their correlation with DNA adducts in female breast tissue', *Mutagenesis* (2009); 24(2): 127–32.

Genkinger JM, Koushik A, 'Meat consumption and cancer risk', *PLOS Medicine* (2007); 4(12): e345.

Block G, Patterson B, Subar A, 'Fruit, vegetables, and cancer prevention: a review of the epidemiological evidence', *Nutrition and Cancer* (1992); 18(1): 1–29.

Wang H, Khor TO, Shu L, *et al.*, 'Plants vs. cancer: a review on natural phytochemicals in preventing and treating cancers and their durability', *Anti-Cancer Agents in Medicinal Chemistry* (2012); 12(10): 1281–1305.

Edenharder R, Sager JW, Glatt H, Muckel E, Platt KL, 'Protection by beverages, fruits, vegetables, herbs, and flavonoids against genotoxicity of 2-acetylaminofluorene and 2-amino-1-methyl-6-phenylimidazo[4,5-b]pyridine (PhIP) in metabolically competent V79 cells', *Mutation Research* (2002); 521(1–2): 57–72.

Weroha SJ, Haluska P, 'The insulin-like growth factor system in cancer', *Endocrinology and Metabolism Clinics of North America* (2012); 41(2): 335–vi.

Jee SH, Kim HJ, Lee J, 'Obesity, insulin resistance and cancer risk', *Yonsei Medical Journal* (2005); 46(4): 449–55.

Grimberg A, 'Mechanisms by which IGF-I may promote cancer', *Cancer Biology & Therapy* (2003); 2(6): 630–35.

Pasanisi P, Bruno E, Venturelli E, *et al.*, 'A

Dietary Intervention to Lower Serum Levels of IGF-I in BRCA Mutation Carriers', *Cancers* (2018); 10(9): 309.

Giovannucci E, 'Insulin, insulin-like growth factors and colon cancer: a review of the evidence', *The Journal of Nutrition* (2001); 131(11): 3109S–20S.

Wolk A, Mantzoros CS, Andersson S-O, Bergstrom R, Signorello LB, Lagiou P, Adami H-O, Trichopoulos D, 'Insulin-like growth factor 1 and prostate cancer risk: a population-based, case-control study', *Journal of the National Cancer Institute* (1998); 90: 911–15.

Chan JM, Stampfer MK, Giovannucci E, Gann PH, Ma J, Wilkinson P, Hennekens CH, Pollak M, 'Plasma insulin-like growth factor-I and prostate cancer risk: a prospective study', *Science* (1998); 279: 563–66.

Rahmani J, Kord Varkaneh H, Clark C, *et al.*, 'The influence of fasting and energy restricting diets on IGF-1 levels in humans: A systematic review and meta-analysis', *Ageing Research Reviews* (2019); 53: 100910.

Williams GP, 'The role of oestrogen in the pathogenesis of obesity, type 2 diabetes, breast cancer and prostate disease', *European Journal of Cancer Prevention* (2010); 19(4): 256–71.

Malekinejad H, Rezabakhsh A, 'Hormones in Dairy Foods and Their Impact on Public Health – A Narrative Review Article', *Iranian Journal of Public Health* (2015); 44(6): 742–58.

Yang CZ, Yaniger SI, Jordan VC, Klein DJ, Bittner GD, 'Most plastic products release estrogenic chemicals: a potential health problem that can be solved', *Environmental Health Perspectives* (2011); 119(7): 989–96.

Ward MH, Cross AJ, Abnet CC, Sinha R, Markin RS, Weisenburger DD, 'Heme iron from meat and risk of adenocarcinoma of the esophagus and stomach', *European Journal of Cancer Prevention* (2012); 21(2): 134–38.

Cross A, J., Pollock, JRA, 'Haem, not Protein or Inorganic Iron, Is Responsible for Endogenous Intestinal N-Nitrosation Arising from Red Meat', *Cancer Research* (2003); 63(10): 2358–60.

genannt Bonsmann SS, Walczyk T, Renggli S, Hurrell RF, 'Oxalic acid does not influence nonhaem iron absorption in humans: a comparison of kale and spinach meals', *European Journal of Clinical Nutrition* (2008); 62(3): 336–41.

Hallberg L, Brune M, Rossander L, 'The role of vitamin C in iron absorption', *International Journal for Vitamin and Nutrition Resesearch* (1989); 30: 103–8.

IARC Monographs on the Evaluation of Carcinogenic Risks to Humans, WHO Press, Online pub, March 2018 No. 114.

SACN Iron and Health Report.

William J Ripple, Christopher Wolf, Thomas M Newsome, Phoebe Barnard, William R Moomaw, 'World Scientists' Warning of a Climate Emergency', *BioScience* (2020); 70(1): 8–12.

Orlich MJ, Singh PN, Sabaté J, *et al.*, 'Vegetarian dietary patterns and mortality in Adventist Health Study 2', *JAMA Internal Medicine* (2013); 173(13): 1230–38.

Tong Tammy Y N, Appleby Paul N, Bradbury Kathryn E, Perez-Cornago Aurora, Travis Ruth C, Clarke Robert *et al.,* 'Risks of ischaemic heart disease and stroke in meat eaters, fish eaters, and vegetarians over 18 years of follow-up: results from the prospective EPIC-Oxford study', *BMJ* (2019); 366: l4897.

Verhoeven DT, Goldbohm RA, van Poppel G, Verhagen H, van den Brandt PA,

'Epidemiological studies on brassica vegetables and cancer risk', *Cancer Epidemiology, Biomarkers & Prevention* (1996); 5(9): 733–48.

Chan CW, Lee PH, 'Association between dietary fibre intake with cancer and all-cause mortality among 15 740 adults: the National Health and Nutrition Examination Survey III', *Journal of Human Nutrition and Dietetics* (2016); 29(5): 633–42.

Masrul M, Nindrea RD, 'Dietary Fibre Protective against Colorectal Cancer Patients in Asia: A Meta-Analysis', *Open Access Macedonian Journal of Medical Sciences* (2019); 7(10): 1723–27. doi: 10.3889/oamjms.2019.265.

Chen S, Chen Y, Ma S, *et al.*, 'Dietary fibre intake and risk of breast cancer: A systematic review and meta-analysis of epidemiological studies', *Oncotarget* (2016); 7(49): 80980–89.

Blackburn GL, Wang KA, 'Dietary fat reduction and breast cancer outcome: results from the Women's Intervention Nutrition'.

Barrera S, Demark-Wahnefried W, 'Nutrition during and after cancer therapy', *Oncology* (2009); 23(2 Suppl Nurse Ed): 15–21.

Sagar SM, Yance D, Wong RK, 'Natural health products that inhibit angiogenesis: a potential source for investigational new agents to treat cancer – Part 1', *Current Oncology* (2006); 13(1): 14–26.

Fiolet T, Srour B, Sellem L, *et al.*, 'Consumption of ultra-processed foods and cancer risk: results from NutriNet-Santé prospective cohort', *BMJ* (2018); 360: k322.

Li Y, Schoufour J, Wang DD, *et al.*, 'Healthy lifestyle and life expectancy free of cancer, cardiovascular disease, and type 2 diabetes: prospective cohort study', *BMJ* (2020); 368: l6669.

Anne-Claire Vergnaud, Dora Romaguera,

Petra H Peeters, *et al.*, 'Adherence to the World Cancer Research Fund/American Institute for Cancer Research guidelines and risk of death in Europe: results from the European Prospective Investigation into Nutrition and Cancer cohort study', *The American Journal of Clinical Nutrition* (2013); 97(5): 1107–20.

Erren TC, Falaturi P, Morfeld P, Knauth P, Reiter RJ, Piekarski C, 'Shift work and cancer: the evidence and the challenge', *Deutsches Ärzteblatt Int.* (2010); 107(38): 657–62.

Hardell L, Carlberg M, Söderqvist F, Mild KH, 'Case-control study of the association between malignant brain tumours diagnosed between 2007 and 2009 and mobile and cordless phone use', *International Journal of Oncology* (2013); 43(6): 1833–45.

Zhao L, Liu X, Wang C, *et al.*, 'Magnetic fields exposure and childhood leukemia risk: a meta-analysis based on 11,699 cases and 13,194 controls', *Leukemia Research* (2014); 38(3): 269–74.

Zhao G, Lin X, Zhou M, Zhao J, 'Relationship between exposure to extremely low-frequency electromagnetic fields and breast cancer risk: a meta-analysis', *European Journal of Gynaecological Oncology* (2014); 35(3): 264–69.

Hardell L, 'World Health Organization, radiofrequency radiation and health – a hard nut to crack (Review)', *International Journal of Oncology* (2017); 51(2): 405–13.

European Parliamentary Research Service Briefing Document: 'Effects of 5G wireless communication on human health'. Published March 2020.

Simkó M, Mattsson MO, '5G Wireless Communication and Health Effects-A Pragmatic Review Based on Available Studies Regarding 6 to 100 GHz', *International Journal of Environmental Research and Public Health*

(2019); 16(18): 3406.

Moreno-Smith M, Lutgendorf SK, Sood AK, 'Impact of stress on cancer metastasis', *Future Oncology* (2010); 6(12): 1863–81.

Maunsell E, Brisson J, Deschenes L, 'Social support and survival among women with breast cancer', *Cancer* (1995); 76(4): 631–37.

DIABETES DISCOVERIES

Qian F, Liu G, Hu FB, Bhupathiraju SN, Sun Q, 'Association Between Plant-Based Dietary Patterns and Risk of Type 2 Diabetes: A Systematic Review and Meta-analysis', *JAMA Internal Medicine* (2019); 179(10): 1335–44.

Al-Goblan AS, Al-Alfi MA, Khan MZ, 'Mechanism linking diabetes mellitus and obesity', *Diabetes, Metabolic Syndrome and Obesity* (2014); 7: 587–91.

Chia JSJ, McRae JL, Kukuljan S, *et al.*, 'A1 beta-casein milk protein and other environmental pre-disposing factors for type 1 diabetes', *Nutrition & Diabetes* (2017); 7(5): e274.

Adler K, Mueller DB, Achenbach P, *et al.*, 'Insulin autoantibodies with high affinity to the bovine milk protein alpha casein', *Clinical and Experimental Immunology* (2011); 164(1): 42–9.

Vaarala O, Ilonen J, Ruohtula T, *et al.*, 'Removal of Bovine Insulin From Cow's Milk Formula and Early Initiation of Beta-Cell Autoimmunity in the FINDIA Pilot Study', *Archives of Pediatrics and Adolescent Medicine* (2012); 166(7): 608–14.

Chia, J.S.J., McRae, J.L.,Enjapoori, A.K., Lefèvre, C.M., Kukuljan, S., Dwyer, K.M., 'Dietary Cows' Milk Protein A1 Beta-Casein Increases the Incidence of T1D in NOD Mice', *Nutrients* (2018); 10: 1291.

Anderson J W, Ward K, 'High-carbohydrate, high-fiber diets for insulin-treated men with diabetes mellitus', *The American Journal of Clinical Nutrition* (1979).

Ley SH, Hamdy O, Mohan V, *et al.*, 'Prevention and management of type 2 diabetes: dietary components and nutritional strategies', *The Lancet* (2014); 383: 1999–2007.

Ye EQ, Chacko SA, Chou EL, *et al.*, 'Greater whole-grain intake is associated with lower risk of type 2 diabetes, cardiovascular disease, and weight gain', *The Journal of Nutrition* (2012); 142: 1304–13.

Cooper AJ, Forouhi NG, Ye Z, *et al.*, 'Fruit and vegetable intake and type 2 diabetes: EPIC-InterAct prospective study and meta-analysis', *European Journal of Clinical Nutrition* (2012); 66: 1082–92.

Rizkalla SW, Bellisle F, Slama G, 'Health benefits of low glycaemic index foods, such as pulses, in diabetic patients and healthy individuals', *British Journal of Nutrition* (2002); 88(Suppl 3): S255–S262.

Qian F, Liu G, Hu FB, Bhupathiraju SN, Sun Q, 'Association Between Plant-Based Dietary Patterns and Risk of Type 2 Diabetes: A Systematic Review and Meta-analysis', *JAMA Internal Medicine* (2019); 179(10): 1335–44.

McMacken M, Shah S, 'A plant-based diet for the prevention and treatment of type 2 diabetes', *Journal of Geriatric Cardiology* (2017); 14(5): 342–54.

Kahleova H, Fleeman R, Hlozkova A, Holubkov R, Barnard ND, 'A plant-based diet in overweight individuals in a 16-week randomized clinical trial: metabolic benefits of plant protein', *Nutrition & Diabetes* (2018); 8(1): 58. doi: 10.1038/s41387-018-0067-4.

Campmans-Kuijpers MJ, Sluijs I, Nothlings U, *et al.*, 'Isocaloric substitution of carbohydrates with protein: the association with weight change and mortality among patients with type 2 diabetes', *Cardiovascular Diabetology* (2015); 14: 39.

Kahleova H, Matoulek M, Malinska H, *et al.*, 'Vegetarian diet improves insulin resistance and oxidative stress markers more than conventional diet in subjects with type 2 diabetes', *Diabetic Medicine* (2011); 28: 549–59.

Sargrad KR, Homko C, Mozzoli M, *et al.*, 'Effect of high protein vs high carbohydrate intake on insulin sensitivity, body weight, hemoglobin A1c, and blood pressure in patients with type 2 diabetes mellitus', *Journal of the American Dietetic Association* (2005); 105: 573–80.

Trapp CB, Barnard ND, 'Usefulness of vegetarian and vegan diets for treating type 2 diabetes', *Current Diabetes Reports* (2010); 10: 152–58.

Goff L M, Bell J D, So P W, Dornhorst A, Frost G S, 'Veganism and its relationship with insulin resistance and intramyocellular lipid', *European Journal of Clinical Nutrition* (2005); 59(2): 291–98.

Alferink, L.J.M., Erler, N.S., de Knegt, R.J. *et al.*, 'Adherence to a plant-based, high-fibre dietary pattern is related to regression of non-alcoholic fatty liver disease in an elderly population', *European Journal of Epidemiology* (2020).

Ward GM, Simpson RW, Simpson HC, Naylor BA, Mann JI, Turner RC, 'Insulin receptor binding increased by high carbohydrate low fat diet in non-insulin-dependent diabetics', *European Journal of Clinical Investigation* (1982); 12(2): 93–6.

Boden G, 'Fatty acid-induced inflammation and insulin resistance in skeletal muscle and liver', *Current Diabetes Reports* (2006); 6(3): 177–81.

Zhang L, Han L, He J, Lv J, Pan R, Lv T, 'A high serum-free fatty acid level is associated with cancer', *Journal of Cancer Research and Clinical Oncology* (2020); 146(3): 705–10.

Yoshikawa H, Tajiri Y, Sako Y, Hashimoto T, Umeda F, Nawata H, 'Effects of free fatty acids on beta-cell functions: a possible involvement of peroxisome proliferator-activated receptors alpha or pancreatic/duodenal homeobox', *Metabolism* (2001); 50(5): 613–18.

J W Anderson, K Ward, 'High-carbohydrate, high-fiber diets for insulin-treated men with diabetes mellitus', *The American Journal of Clinical Nutrition* (1979); 32(11): 2312–21.

Rizkalla SW, Bellisle F, Slama G, 'Health benefits of low glycaemic index foods, such as pulses, in diabetic patients and healthy individuals', *British Journal of Nutrition* (2002); 88(Suppl 3): S255–S262.

Tarini J, Wolever TM, 'The fermentable fibre inulin increases postprandial serum short-chain fatty acids and reduces free-fatty acids and ghrelin in healthy subject', *Applied Physiology, Nutrition and Metabolism* (2010); 35(1): 9–16.

Pingitore A, Chambers ES, Hill T, *et al.*, 'The diet-derived short chain fatty acid propionate improves beta-cell function in humans and stimulates insulin secretion from human islets in vitro', *Diabetes, Obesity and Metabolism* (2017); 19(2): 257–65.

Thompson SV, Winham DM, Hutchins AM, 'Bean and rice meals reduce postprandial glycemic response in adults with type 2 diabetes: a cross-over study', *Nutrition Journal* (2012); 11: 23.

Noto H, Goto A, Tsujimoto T, Noda M, 'Low-carbohydrate diets and all-cause mortality: a systematic review and meta-analysis of observational studies', *PLOS One* (2013); 8(1): e55030.

Foster GD, Wyatt HR, Hill JO, *et al.*, 'A randomized trial of a low-carbohydrate diet for obesity', *The New England Journal of Medicine* (2003); 348(21): 2082–90.

Hall KD, Chen KY, Guo J, *et al.,* 'Energy expenditure and body composition changes after an isocaloric ketogenic diet in overweight and obese men', *American Journal of Clinical Nutrition* (2016); 104(2): 324–33.

Schwingshackl L, Hoffmann G, 'Low-carbohydrate diets and cardiovascular risk factors', *Obesity Reviews* (2013); 14(2): 183–84.

Merino J, *et al.,* 'Negative effects of a low carbohydrate high protein high fat diet on small peripheral artery reactivity in patients with increased cardiovascular risk', *British Journal of Community Nursing* (2012).

Fleming RM, 'The effect of high-protein diets on coronary blood flow', *Angiology* (2000); 51(10): 817–26.

Bolla AM, Caretto A, Laurenzi A, Scavini M, Piemonti L, 'Low-Carb and Ketogenic Diets in Type 1 and Type 2 Diabetes', *Nutrients* (2019); 11(5): 962.

Lu M, Wan Y, Yang B, Huggins CE, Li D, 'Effects of low-fat compared with high-fat diet on cardiometabolic indicators in people with overweight and obesity without overt metabolic disturbance: a systematic review and meta-analysis of randomised controlled trials', *British Journal of Nutrition* (2018); 119(1): 96–108.

Dinu M, Abbate R, Gensini GF, Casini A, Sofi F, 'Vegetarian, vegan diets and multiple health outcomes: A systematic review with meta-analysis of observational studies', *Critical Reviews in Food Science and Nutrition* (2017); 57(17): 3640–49.

Kempner W, Peschel RL, Schlayer C, 'Effect of rice diet on diabetes mellitus associated with vascular disease', *Postgraduate Medicine* (1958); 24: 359–71.

Dunaief D M, Fuhrman J, Dunaief J L, Ying G, 'Glycemic and cardiovascular parameters improved in type 2 diabetes with the high nutrient density (HND) diet', *Open Journal of Preventive Medicine* (2012); 2(3): 364.

Tonstad S, Butler T, Yan R, Fraser GE, 'Type of vegetarian diet, body weight, and prevalence of type 2 diabetes', *Diabetes Care* (2009); 32(5): 791–96. doi: 10.2337/dc08-1886.

RESET YOUR SKIN

Cordain L, Lindeberg S, Hurtado M, Hill K, Eaton SB, Brand-Miller J, 'Acne vulgaris: a disease of Western civilization', *Archives of Dermatology* (2002); 138(12): 1584–90.

Smith RN, Mann NJ, Braue A, Mäkeläinen H, Varigos GA, 'A low-glycemic-load diet improves symptoms in acne vulgaris patients: a randomized controlled trial', *American Journal of Clinical Nutrition* (2007); 86(1): 107–15.

Melnik B C, 'Diet in acne: Further evidence for the role of nutrient signalling in acne pathogenesis', *Acta Dermato-Venereologica* (2012); 92(3): 228–1.

B C Melnik, 'Dietary intervention in acne: Attenuation of increased mTORC1 signaling promoted by Western diet', *Dermato-Endocrinology* (2012); 4(1): 20–32.

Danby F W, 'Turning acne on/off via mTORC1', *Experimental Dermatology* (2013); 22(7): 505–06.

Melnik B C, John S M, Carrera-Bastos P, Cordain L, 'The impact of cow's milk-mediated mTORC1-signaling in the initiation and progression of prostate cancer', *Nutrition and Metabolism* (2012); 9(1): 74.

Mirzaei H, Suarez JA, Longo VD, 'Protein and amino acid restriction, aging and disease: from yeast to humans', *Trends in Endocrinology and Metabolism* (2014); 25(11): 558–66.

Block SG, Valins WE, Caperton CV, Viera MH, Amini S, Berman B, 'Exacerbation of facial acne vulgaris after consuming pure chocolate', *Journal of the American Academy of Dermatology* (2011); 65(4): e114–5.

Vongraviopap S, Asawanonda P, 'Dark chocolate exacerbates acne', Inteernational Journal of Dermatology (2016); 55(5): 587–91.

Pierre Dougan and Naser Rafikhah, 'Dark and White Chocolate Consumption and Acne Vulgaris: A Case-Control Study', *Asian Journal of Clinical Nutrition* (2014); 6: 35–40.

Caperton C, Block S, Viera M, Keri J, Berman B, 'Double-blind, Placebo-controlled Study Assessing the Effect of Chocolate Consumption in Subjects with a History of Acne Vulgaris', *The Journal of Clinical and Aesthetic Dermatology* (2014); 7(5): 19–23.

Kucharska A, Szmurło A, Sińska B, 'Significance of diet in treated and untreated acne vulgaris', *Postepy Dermatologii I Alergologii* (2016); 33(2): 81–6.

Zhang B, Zhao Q, Guo W, Bao W, Wang X, 'Association of whole grain intake with all-cause, cardiovascular, and cancer mortality: a systematic review and dose-response meta-analysis from prospective cohort studies', *European Journal of Clinical Nutrition* (2018); 72(1): 57–65.

Carey OJ, *et al.*, 'The effect of lifestyle on wheeze, atopy, and bronchial hyper-reactivity in Asian and white children', *American Journal of Respiratory and Critical Care Medicine* (1996); 154: 537.

Zhang A, Silverberg JI, 'Association of atopic dermatitis with being overweight and obese: a systematic review and metaanalysis', *JAAD* (2015); 72: 606.

Wright RJ, Cohen RT, Cohen S, 'The impact of stress on the development and expression of atopy', *Current Opinion in Allergy and Clinical Immunology* (2005); 5(1): 23–9.

Liezmann C, Klapp B, Peters EM, 'Stress, atopy and allergy: A re-evaluation from a psychoneuroimmunologic persepective', *Dermato-Endocrinology* (2011); 3(1): 37–40.

Park S, Choi HS, Bae JH, 'Instant noodles, processed food intake, and dietary pattern are associated with atopic dermatitis in an adult population', *Asia Pacific Journal of Clinical Nutrition* (2016); 25: 602.

Cepeda AM, *et al.*, 'A Traditional Diet Is Associated with a Reduced Risk of Eczema and Wheeze in Colombian Children', *Nutrients* (2015); 7: 5098.

Tanaka T, *et al.*, 'Vegetarian diet ameliorates symptoms of atopic dermatitis through reduction of the number of peripheral eosinophils and of PGE2 synthesis by monocytes', *Journal of Physiological Anthropology and Applied Human Science* (2001); 20: 353.

HORMONES AND HEALTH

Day FR, Elks CE, Murray A, Ong KK, Perry JR, 'Puberty timing associated with diabetes, cardiovascular disease and also diverse health outcomes in men and women: the UK Biobank study', *Scientific Reports* (2015); 5: 11208.

Lazzeri G, Tosti C, Pammolli A, *et al.*, 'Overweight and lower age at menarche: evidence from the Italian HBSC cross-sectional survey', *BMC Women's Health* (2018); 18(1): 168.

Trichopoulos D, MacMahon B, Cole P, 'Menopause and breast cancer risk', *Journal of the National Cancer Institute* (1972); 48(3): 605–13.

Hershcopf RJ, Bradlow HL, 'Obesity, diet, endogenous estrogens, and the risk of hormone-sensitive cancer', *American Journal of Clinical*

Nutrition (1987); 45(1 Suppl): 283–89.

Meier R, Beglinger C, Dederding JP, *et al.*, 'Influence of age, gender, hormonal status and smoking habits on colonic transit time', *Neurogastroenterology & Motility* (1995); 7(4): 235–38.

Wang Z, Liu H, Liu S, 'Low-Dose Bisphenol A Exposure: A Seemingly Instigating Carcinogenic Effect on Breast Cancer', *Advanced Science* (2016); 4(2): 1600248.

Gao H, Yang BJ, Li N, *et al.*, 'Bisphenol A and hormone-associated cancers: current progress and perspectives', *Medicine (Baltimore)* (2015); 94(1): e211.

Mnif W, Hassine AI, Bouaziz A, Bartegi A, Thomas O, Roig B, 'Effect of endocrine disruptor pesticides: a review', *International Journal of Environmental Research and Public Health* (2011); 8(6): 2265–303.

Braun JM, Sathyanarayana S, Hauser R, 'Phthalate exposure and children's health', *Current Opinion in Pediatrics* (2013); 25(2): 247–54.

Kay VR, Chambers C, Foster WG, 'Reproductive and developmental effects of phthalate diesters in females', *Critical Reviews in Toxicology* (2013); 43(3): 200–19.

Hsieh TH, Tsai CF, Hsu CY, *et al.*, 'Phthalates induce proliferation and invasiveness of estrogen receptor-negative breast cancer through the AhR/HDAC6/c-Myc signaling pathway', *The FASEB Journal* (2012); 26(2): 778–87.

Barnard ND1, Scialli AR, Hurlock D, Bertron P, 'Diet and sex-hormone binding globulin, dysmenorrhea, and premenstrual symptoms. Randomized controlled trial', *Obstetrics & Gynecology* (2000); 95(2): 245–50.

Lasco A, Catalano A, Benvenga S, 'Improvement of Primary Dysmenorrhea Caused by a Single Oral Dose of Vitamin D: Results of a Randomized, Double-blind, Placebo-Controlled Study', *Archives of Internal Medicine* (2012); 172(4): 366–67.

Rahnama P, Montazeri A, Huseini HF, Kianbakht S, Naseri M, 'Effect of Zingiber officinale R. rhizomes (ginger) on pain relief in primary dysmenorrhea: a placebo randomized trial', *BMC Complementary and Alternative Medicine* (2012); 12: 92.

Ozgoli G, Goli M, Moatar F, 'Comparison of effects of ginger, mefenamic acid, and ibuprofen on pain in women with primary dysmenorrhea', *The Journal of Alternative and Complementary Medicine* (2009); 15: 129–32.

Karamali M, Kashanian M, Alaeinasab S, Asemi Z, 'The effect of dietary soy intake on weight loss, glycaemic control, lipid profiles and biomarkers of inflammation and oxidative stress in women with polycystic ovary syndrome: a randomised clinical trial', *Journal of Human Nutrition and Dietetics* (2018); 31(4): 533–43.

Khani B, Mehrabian F, Khalesi E, Eshraghi A, 'Effect of soy phytoestrogen on metabolic and hormonal disturbance of women with polycystic ovary syndrome', *Journal of Research in Medical Sciences* (2011); 16(3): 297–302.

Yamamoto A, Harris HR, Vitonis AF, *et al.*, 'A prospective cohort study of meat and fish consumption and endometriosis risk', *American Journal of Obstetrics and Gynecology* (2018); 219: 178.e1–10.

Bradley EL, Burden RA, Bentayeb K, *et al.*, 'Exposure to phthalic acid, phthalate diesters and phthalate monoesters from foodstuffs: UK total diet study results', *Food Additives and Contaminants: Part A Chem Anal Control Expo Risk Assess.* (2013); 30(4): 735–42.

Schecter A, Lorber M, Guo Y, *et al.*, 'Phthalate concentrations and dietary exposure from food purchased in New York State', *Environmental Health Perspectives* (2013); 121(4): 473–94.

Diamanti-Kandarakis E, Bourguignon JP, Giudice LC, *et al.*, 'Endocrine-disrupting chemicals: an Endocrine Society scientific statement', *Endocrine Reviews* (2009); 30(4): 293–342.

Katz TA, Yang Q, Treviño LS, Walker CL, Al-Hendy A, 'Endocrine-disrupting chemicals and uterine fibroids', *Fertility and Sterility* (2016); 106(4): 967–77.

Parazzini, Fabio, Di Martino, Mirella, Candiani, Massimo & Viganò, Paola, 'Dietary Components and Uterine Leiomyomas: A Review of Published Data', *Nutrition and Cancer* (2015); 67(4): 569–79.

Takala H, Yang Q, El Razek AMA, Ali M, Al-Hendy A, 'Alcohol Consumption and Risk of Uterine Fibroids', *Current Molecular Medicine* (2020); 20(4): 247–58.

Qin H, Lin Z, Vásquez E, Xu L, 'The association between chronic psychological stress and uterine fibroids risk: A meta-analysis of observational studies', *Stress Health* (2019); 35(5): 585–94.

Lock M, 'Menopause: lessons from anthropology', *Psychosomatic Medicine* (1998); 60(4): 410–19.

Nagata C, Takatsuka N, Kowakami N, Shimuzu H, 'Soy product intake and hot flashes in Japanese women: results from a community based prospective study', *American Journal of Epidemiology* (2001); 153: 790–93.

Nagata C, Shimizu H, Takami R, Hayashi M, Takeda N, Yasuda K, 'Hot flashes and other menopausal symptoms in relation to soy product intake in Japanese Women', *Climacteric* (1999); 2: 6–12.

Chen WY, Rosner B, Hankinson SE, Colditz GA, Willett WC, 'Moderate alcohol consumption during adult life, drinking patterns, and breast cancer risk', *JAMA* (2011); 306(17): 1884–90.

Bonde JP, 'Male reproductive organs are at risk from environmental hazards', *Asian Journal of Andrology* (2010); 12(2): 152–56.

Hu GX, Lian QQ, Ge RS, Hardy DO, Li XK, 'Phthalate-induced testicular dysgenesis syndrome: Leydig cell influence', *Trends in Endocrinology & Metabolism* (2009); 20(3): 139–45.

Ricci E, Al Beitawi S, Cipriani S, *et al.*, 'Semen quality and alcohol intake: a systematic review and meta-analysis', *Reproductive BioMedicine Online* (2017); 34(1): 38–47.

Mendiola, Jaime *et al.*, 'Food intake and its relationship with semen quality: a case-control study', *Fertility and Sterility* 91(3): 812–18.

Attaman, Jill A., Toth, Thomas L., Furtado ,Jeremy, Campos, Hannia, Hauser, Russ, Chavarro, Jorge. E., 'Dietary fat and semen quality among men attending a fertility clinic', *Human Reproduction* (2012); 27(5): 1466–74.

Cito G, Cocci A, Micelli E, *et al.*, 'Vitamin D and Male Fertility: An Updated Review', *The World Journal of Men's Health* (2020); 38(2): 164–77.

Esposito K, Giugliano F, Di Palo C, *et al.*, 'Effect of lifestyle changes on erectile dysfunction in obese men: a randomized controlled trial', *JAMA* (2004); 291(24): 2978–84.

Paterni I, Granchi C, Katzenellenbogen JA, Minutolo F, 'Estrogen receptors alpha (ERβ) and beta (ERβ): subtype-selective ligands and clinical potential', *Steroids* (2014); 90: 13–29.

Mahmoud AM, Al-Alem U, Ali MM, Bosland MC, 'Genistein increases estrogen receptor beta expression in prostate cancer via reducing its promoter methylation', *The Journal of Steroid Biochemistry and Molecular Biology* (2015); 152: 62–75.

D. L. Alekel, A. S. Germain, C. T. Peterson, K. B. Hanson, J. W. Stewart, and T. Toda, 'Isoflavone-rich soy protein isolate attenuates bone loss in the lumbar spine of perimenopausal women', *American Journal of Clinical Nutrition* (2000); 72(3): 844–52.

Castro SI, Berthiaume R, Robichaud A, Lacasse P, 'Effects of iodine intake and teat-dipping practices on milk iodine concentrations in dairy cows', *Journal of Dairy Science* (2012); 95(1): 213–20.

Tonstad S, Nathan E, Oda K, Fraser G, 'Vegan diets and hypothyroidism', *Nutrients* (2013); 5(11): 4642–52. P

Manzel A, Muller DN, Hafler DA, Erdman SE, Linker RA, Kleinewietfeld M, 'Role of "Western diet" in inflammatory autoimmune diseases', *Current Allergy and Asthma Reports* (2014); 14(1): 404.

A HEALTHY GUT

Hills RD Jr, Pontefract BA, Mishcon HR, Black CA, Sutton SC, Theberge CR, 'Gut Microbiome: Profound Implications for Diet and Disease', *Nutrients* (2019); 11(7): 1613.

Zinöcker MK, Lindseth IA, 'The Western Diet-Microbiome-Host Interaction and Its Role in Metabolic Disease', *Nutrients* (2018); 10(3): 365.

Tomova A, Bukovsky I, Rembert E, *et al.*, 'The Effects of Vegetarian and Vegan Diets on Gut Microbiota', *Frontiers in Nutrition* (2019); 6: 47.

Najjar RS, Feresin RG, 'Plant-Based Diets in the Reduction of Body Fat: Physiological Effects and Biochemical Insights', *Nutrients* (2019); 11(11): 2712.

Murphy EA, Velazquez KT, Herbert KM, 'Influence of high-fat diet on gut microbiota: a driving force for chronic disease risk', *Current Opinion in Clinical Nutrition & Metabolic Care* (2015); 18(5): 515–20.

Kanitsoraphan C, Rattanawong P, Charoensri S, Senthong V, 'Trimethylamine N-Oxide and Risk of Cardiovascular Disease and Mortality', *Current Nutrition Reports* (2018); 7(4): 207–13.

Tang WH, Wang Z, Kennedy DJ, *et al.*, 'Gut microbiota-dependent trimethylamine N-oxide (TMAO) pathway contributes to both development of renal insufficiency and mortality risk in chronic kidney disease', *Circulation Research* (2015); 116(3): 448–55.

Koeth RA, Wang Z, Levison BS, *et al.*, 'Intestinal microbiota metabolism of L-carnitine, a nutrient in red meat, promotes atherosclerosis', *Nature Medicine* (2013); 19(5): 576–85.

Corrêa-Oliveira R, Fachi JL, Vieira A, Sato FT, Vinolo MA, 'Regulation of immune cell function by short-chain fatty acids', *Clinical & Translational Immunology* (2016); 5(4): e73.

Yang Y, Zhao LG, Wu QJ, Ma X, Xiang YB, 'Association between dietary fiber and lower risk of all-cause mortality: a meta-analysis of cohort studies', *American Journal of Epidemiology* (2015); 181(2): 83–91.

Yoon MY, Yoon SS, 'Disruption of the Gut Ecosystem by Antibiotics', *Yonsei Medical Journal* (2018); 59(1): 4–12.

Kelesidis T, Pothoulakis C, 'Efficacy and safety of the probiotic Saccharomyces boulardii for the prevention and therapy of gastrointestinal disorders', *Therapeutic Advances in Gastroenterology* (2012); 5(2): 111–25.

Suez J, Zmora N, Zilberman-Schapira G, *et al.*, 'Post-Antibiotic Gut Mucosal Microbiome Reconstitution Is Impaired by Probiotics and

Improved by Autologous FMT', *Cell* (2018); 174(6): 1406–23. e16.

Martin MJ, Thottathil SE, Newman TB, 'Antibiotics Overuse in Animal Agriculture: A Call to Action for Health Care Providers', *American Journal of Public Health* (2015); 105(12): 2409–10. doi: 10.2105/AJPH.2015.302870.

Aldoori WH, Giovannucci EL, Rockett HR, Sampson L, Rimm EB, Willett WC, 'A prospective study of dietary fiber types and symptomatic diverticular disease in men', *The Journal of Nutrition* (1998); 128(4): 714–19.

Cummings JH, Engineer A, 'Denis Burkitt and the origins of the dietary fibre hypothesis', *Nutrition Research Reviews* (2018); 31(1): 1–15.

Rizzello F, Spisni E, Giovanardi E, *et al.*, 'Implications of the Westernized Diet in the Onset and Progression of IBD', *Nutrients* (2019); 11(5): 1033.

Hou JK, Abraham B, El-Serag H, 'Dietary intake and risk of developing inflammatory bowel disease: a systematic review of the literature', *The American Journal of Gastroenterology* (2011); 106(4): 563–73.

Haskey N, Gibson DL, 'An Examination of Diet for the Maintenance of Remission in Inflammatory Bowel Disease', *Nutrients* (2017); 9(3): 259.

Sandefur K, Kahleova H, Desmond AN, Elfrink E, Barnard ND, 'Crohn's Disease Remission with a Plant-Based Diet: A Case Report', *Nutrients* (2019); 11(6): 1385.

Ananthakrishnan AN, Khalili H, Konijeti GG, *et al.*, 'A prospective study of long-term intake of dietary fiber and risk of Crohn's disease and ulcerative colitis', *Gastroenterology* (2013); 145(5): 970–77.

Preshaw PM, 'Mouthwash use and risk of diabetes', *British Dental Journal* (2018); 225(10): 923–26.

Bondonno C P, Liu A H, Croft K D *et al.*, 'Antibacterial mouthwash blunts oral nitrate reduction and increases blood pressure in treated hypertensive men and women', *American Journal of Hypertension* (2015); 28: 572–75.

Kaczmarek JL, Thompson SV, Holscher HD, 'Complex interactions of circadian rhythms, eating behaviors, and the gastrointestinal microbiota and their potential impact on health', *Nutrition Reviews* (2017); 75(9): 673–82.

Karl JP, Hatch AM, Arcidiacono SM, *et al.*, 'Effects of Psychological, Environmental and Physical Stressors on the Gut Microbiota', *Frontiers in Microbiology* (2018); 9: 2013.

Smith RP, Easson C, Lyle SM, *et al.*, 'Gut microbiome diversity is associated with sleep physiology in humans', *PLOS One* (2019); 14(10): e0222394.

Monda V, Villano I, Messina A, *et al.*, 'Exercise Modifies the Gut Microbiota with Positive Health Effects', *Oxidative Medicine and Cellular Longevity* (2017); 2017: 3831972.

Rogers MAM, Aronoff DM, 'The influence of non-steroidal anti-inflammatory drugs on the gut microbiome', *Clinical Microbiology and Infection* (2016); 22(2): 178.e1–178.e9.

Cornish JA, Tan E, Simillis C, Clark SK, Teare J, Tekkis PP, 'The risk of oral contraceptives in the etiology of inflammatory bowel disease: a meta-analysis', *The American Journal of Gastroenterology* (2008); 103(9): 2394–400.

Chassaing B, Van de Wiele T, De Bodt J, Marzorati M, Gewirtz AT, 'Dietary emulsifiers directly alter human microbiota composition and gene expression ex vivo potentiating intestinal inflammation', *Gut* (2017); 66(8): 1414–27.

Ruiz-Ojeda FJ, Plaza-Díaz J, Sáez-Lara MJ, Gil A, 'Effects of Sweeteners on the Gut Microbiota: A Review of Experimental Studies and Clinical Trials', *Advances in Nutrition* (2019);10(suppl_1): S31–S48.

Collins J, Robinson C, Danhof H, *et al.*, 'Dietary trehalose enhances virulence of epidemic Clostridium difficile', *Nature* (2018); 553(7688): 291–94.

IMMUNITY

Sutliffe JT, Wilson LD, de Heer HD, Foster RL, Carnot MJ, 'C-reactive protein response to a vegan lifestyle intervention', *Complementary Therapies in Medicine* (2015); 23(1): 32–7.

Jaceldo-Siegl K, Haddad E, Knutsen S, *et al.*, 'Lower C-reactive protein and IL-6 associated with vegetarian diets are mediated by BMI', *Nutrition, Metabolism & Cardiovascular Diseases* (2018); 28(8): 787–94.

Haghighatdoost F, Bellissimo N, Totosy de Zepetnek JO, Rouhani MH, 'Association of vegetarian diet with inflammatory biomarkers: a systematic review and meta-analysis of observational studies', *Public Health Nutrition* (2017); 20(15): 2713–21.

Alwarith J, Kahleova H, Rembert E, *et al.*, 'Nutrition Interventions in Rheumatoid Arthritis: The Potential Use of Plant-Based Diets. A Review', *Frontiers in Nutrition* (2019); 6: 141.

David LA, Maurice CF, Carmody RN, *et al.*, 'Diet rapidly and reproducibly alters the human gut microbiome', *Nature* (2014); 505(7484): 559–63.

Horta-Baas G, Romero-Figueroa MDS, Montiel-Jarquín AJ, Pizano-Zárate ML, García-Mena J, Ramírez-Durán N, 'Intestinal Dysbiosis and Rheumatoid Arthritis: A Link between Gut Microbiota and the Pathogenesis of Rheumatoid Arthritis', *Journal of Immunology Research* (2017); 2017: 4835189.

Ratajczak W, Ryl A, Mizerski A, Walczakiewicz K, Sipak O, Laszczyńska M, 'Immunomodulatory potential of gut microbiome-derived short-chain fatty acids (SCFAs)', *Acta Biochimica Polonica* (2019); 66(1): 1–12.

Kjeldsen-Kragh J, Haugen M, Borchgrevink CF, *et al.*, 'Controlled trial of fasting and one-year vegetarian diet in rheumatoid'.

McDougall J, Bruce B, Spiller G, Westerdahl J, McDougall M, 'Effects of a very low-fat, vegan diet in subjects with rheumatoid arthritis', *Journal of Alternative and Complementary Medicine* (2002); 8: 71–5.

Elkan AC, Sjöberg B, Kolsrud B, Ringertz B, Hafström I, Frostegård J, 'Gluten-free vegan diet induces decreased LDL and oxidized LDL levels and raised atheroprotective natural antibodies against phosphorylcholine in patients with rheumatoid arthritis: a randomized study', *Arthritis Research & Therapy* (2008); 10(2): R34.

Alwarith J, Kahleova H, Rembert E, *et al.*, 'Nutrition Interventions in Rheumatoid Arthritis: The Potential Use of Plant-Based Diets. A Review', *Frontiers in Nutrition* (2019); 6: 141.

Constantin MM, Nita IE, Olteanu R, *et al.*, 'Significance and impact of dietary factors on systemic lupus erythematosus pathogenesis', *Experimental and Therapeutic Medicine* (2019); 17(2): 1085–90.

Swank RL, Lerstad O, Strøm A, Backer J, 'Multiple sclerosis in rural Norway its geographic and occupational incidence in relation to nutrition', *New England Journal of Medicine* (1952); 246(19): 722–28.

Ran L, Zhao W, Wang J, *et al.*, 'Extra Dose of Vitamin C Based on a Daily Supplementation

Shortens the Common Cold: A Meta-Analysis of 9 Randomized Controlled Trials', *BioMed Research Interational* (2018); 2018: 1837634.

MASTERING THE BUILDING BLOCKS OF WFPB EATING

Jakobsen MU, O'Reilly EJ, Heitmann BL, *et al*., 'Major types of dietary fat and risk of coronary heart disease: a pooled analysis of 11 cohort studies', *American Journal of Clinical Nutrition* (2009); 89(5): 1425–32.

Farvid MS, Ding M, Pan A, *et al*., 'Dietary linoleic acid and risk of coronary heart disease: a systematic review and meta-analysis of prospective cohort studies', *Circulation* (2014); 130(18): 1568–78.

Mozaffarian D, Micha R, Wallace S, 'Effects on coronary heart disease of increasing polyunsaturated fat in place of saturated fat: a systematic review and meta-analysis of randomized controlled trials', *PLOS Medicine* (2010); 7(3): e1000252.

Zong G, Li Y, Sampson L, *et al*., 'Monounsaturated fats from plant and animal sources in relation to risk of coronary heart disease among US men and women', American Journal of Clinical Nutrition (2018); 107(3): 445–53.

Aune D, Giovannucci E, Boffetta P, *et al*., 'Fruit and vegetable intake and the risk of cardiovascular disease, total cancer and all-cause mortality-a systematic review and dose-response meta-analysis of prospective studies', *International Journal of Epidemiology* (2017); 46(3): 1029–56.

Smith-Spangler, Crystal, Brandeau, Margaret L., Hunter, Grace E., Clay Bavinger, J., *et al*., 'Are Organic Foods Safer or Healthier Than Conventional Alternatives?', *Annals of Internal Medicine* (2012); 157(5): 348–66.

Hoppin JA, Umbach DM, Long S, *et al*., 'Pesticides are Associated with Allergic and Non-Allergic Wheeze among Male Farmers', *Environmental Health Perspectives* (2017); 125(4): 535–43.

Buralli RJ, Dultra AF, Ribeiro H, 'Respiratory and Allergic Effects in Children Exposed to Pesticides – A Systematic Review', *International Journal of Environmental Research and Public Health* (2020); 17(8): 2740.

Hyland, C., Laribi, O., 'Review of take-home pesticide exposure pathway in children living in agricultural areas', *Environmental Research* (2017); 156: 559–70.

Lu, C., Toepel, K., Irish, R., Fenske, R.A., Barr, D.B., Bravo, R, 'Organic diets significantly lower children's dietary exposure to organophosphorus pesticides', *Environmental Health Perspectives* (2006); 114: 260–63.

Marks, A.R., Harley, K., Bradman, A., Kogut, K., Barr, D.B., Johnson, C., Calderon, N., Eskenazi, B., 'Organophosphate pesticide exposure and attention in young Mexican-American children: The CHAMACOS study', *Environmental Health Perspectives* (2010); 118: 1768–74.

Salameh, P.R., Baldi, I., Brochard, P., Raherison, C., Saleh, B.A., Salamon, R., 'Respiratory symptoms in children and exposure to pesticides', *European Respiratory Journal* (2003); 22: 507–12.

Salam, M.T., Li, Y.F., Langholz, B., Gilliland, F.D., 'Early-life environmental risk factors for asthma: Findings from the children's health study', *Environmental Health Perspectives* (2004); 112: 760–65.

Xu, X., Nembhard, W.N., Kan, H., Becker, A., Talbott, E.O., 'Residential pesticide use is associated with children's respiratory symptoms', *Journal of Occupational and Environmental Medicine* (2012); 54: 1281–87.

Raanan, R., Balmes, J.R., Harley, K.G., Gunier, R.B., Magzamen, S., Bradman, A., Eskenazi, B., 'Decreased lung function in 7-year-old children with early-life organophosphate exposure', *Thorax*

(2016); 71: 148–53.

Richardson JR, Roy A, Shalat SL, *et al.*, 'Elevated Serum Pesticide Levels and Risk for Alzheimer Disease, *JAMA Neurology* (2014); 71(3): 284–90.

Zhang, Luoping, Rana, Iemaan, Shaffer, Rachel M., Taioli, Emanuela, Sheppard, Lianne, 'Exposure to glyphosate-based herbicides and risk for non-Hodgkin lymphoma: A meta-analysis and supporting evidence', *Mutation Research/Reviews in Mutation Research* (2019); 781: 186–206.

Zahm SH, Blair A, 'Pesticides and non-Hodgkin's lymphoma', *Cancer Research* (1992); 52(19 Suppl): 5485s–88s.

Pearce N, McLean D, 'Agricultural exposures and non-Hodgkin's lymphoma', *Scandinavian Journal of Work, Environment & Health* (2005); 31(1): 18–27.

Baudry J, Assmann KE, Touvier M, *et al.*, 'Association of frequency of organic food consumption with cancer risk: findings from the NutriNet-Santé Prospective Cohort Study', *JAMA Internale Medicine* [published online October 22, 2018]

Aizen MA, Garibaldi LA, Cunningham SA, Klein AM, 'How much does agriculture depend on pollinators? Lessons from long-term trends in crop production', *Annals of Botany* (2009); 103(9): 1579–88.

Davis DR, Epp MD, Riordan HD, 'Changes in USDA food composition data for 43 garden crops, 1950 to 1999', *Journal of the American College of Nutrition* (2004); 23(6): 669–82.

Loladze, Irakli, 'Hidden shift of the ionome of plants exposed to elevated CO2 depletes minerals at the base of human nutrition', *Ecology, Epidemiology and Global Health* (7 May 2014).

Springmann M, Clark M, Mason-D'Croz D, *et al.*, 'Options for keeping the food system within environmental limits', *Nature* (2018); 562(7728): 519–25.

Kassam, T. Friedrich, Derpsch. R., 'Global spread of Conservation Agriculture', *International Journal of Environmental Studies* (2019); 76(1): 29–51.

Misselwitz B, Butter M, Verbeke K, *et al.*, 'Update on lactose malabsorption and intolerance: pathogenesis, diagnosis and clinical management', *Gut* (2019); 68: 2080–91.

Springmann M, Wiebe K, Mason-D'Croz D, Sulser TB, Rayner M, Scarborough P, 'Health and nutritional aspects of sustainable diet strategies and their association with environmental impacts: a global modelling analysis with country-level detail', *Lancet Planet Health* (2018); 2(10): e451–e461.

Lampe JW, 'Dairy products and cancer', *Journal of the American College of Nutrition* (2011); 30(5 Suppl 1): 464S–70S.

Michaëlsson K, Wolk A, Langenskiöld S, *et al.*, 'Milk intake and risk of mortality and fractures in women and men: cohort studies', *BMJ* (2014); 349: g6015.

Feskanich D, Bischoff-Ferrari HA, Frazier AL, Willett WC, 'Milk consumption during teenage years and risk of hip fractures in older adults', *JAMA Pediatrics* (2014); 168(1): 54–60.

Bo-Htay C, Palee S, Apaijai N, Chattipakorn SC, Chattipakorn N, 'Effects of d-galactose-induced ageing on the heart and its potential interventions', *Journal of Cellular and Molecular Medicine* (2018); 22(3): 1392–1410.

Cramer DW, Greenberg ER, Titus-Ernstoff L, *et al.*, 'A case-control study of galactose consumption and metabolism in relation to ovarian cancer', *Cancer Epidemiology, Biomarkers & Prevention* (2000); 9(1): 95–101.

Cui X, Zuo P, Zhang Q, *et al.*, 'Chronic systemic D-galactose exposure induces memory loss, neurodegeneration, and oxidative damage in mice: protective effects of R-alpha-lipoic acid', *Journal of Neuroscience Research* (2006); 83(8): 1584–90.

Fraser G, Miles F, Orlich M, Jaceldo-Siegl K, Mashchak A, 'Dairy Milk Is Associated with Increased Risk of Breast Cancer in the Adventist Health Study-2 (AHS-2) Cohort (P05-026-19)', *Current Developments in Nutrition* (2019); 3(1): nzz030.P05-026-19.

Song Y, Chavarro JE, Cao Y, *et al.*, 'Whole milk intake is associated with prostate cancer-specific mortality among U.S. male physicians', *Journal of Nutrition* (2013); 143(2): 189–96.

Larsson SC, Orsini N, Wolk A, 'Milk, milk products and lactose intake and ovarian cancer risk: a meta-analysis of epidemiological studies', *International Journal of Cancer* (2006); 118(2): 431–41.

Fairfield KM, Hunter DJ, Colditz GA, *et al.*, 'A prospective study of dietary lactose and ovarian cancer', *International Journal of Cancer* (2004); 110(2): 271–77.

Ji J, Sundquist J, Sundquist K, 'Lactose intolerance and risk of lung, breast and ovarian cancers: aetiological clues from a population-based study in Sweden', *British Journal of Cancer* (2015); 112(1): 149–52.

Naser SA, Ghobrial G, Romero C, Valentine JF, 'Culture of Mycobacterium avium subspecies paratuberculosis from the blood of patients with Crohn's disease', *The Lancet* (2004); 364(9439): 1039–44.

Dow CT, 'Paratuberculosis and Type I diabetes: is this the trigger?', *Medical Hypotheses* (2006); 67(4): 782–85.

Bo M, Erre GL, Bach H, *et al.*, 'PtpA and PknG Proteins Secreted by Mycobacterium avium subsp. paratuberculosis are Recognized by Sera from Patients with Rheumatoid Arthritis: A Case-Control Study', *Journal of Inflammation Research* (2019); 12: 301–08.

Groot MJ, Van't Hooft KE, 'The Hidden Effects of Dairy Farming on Public and Environmental Health in the Netherlands, India, Ethiopia, and Uganda, Considering the Use of Antibiotics and Other Agro-chemicals', *Frontiers in Public Health* (2016); 4: 12.

Chai W, Liebman M, 'Effect of different cooking methods on vegetable oxalate content', *Journal of Agricultural and Food Chemistry* (2005); 53(8): 3027–30.

Vanga SK, Raghavan V, 'How well do plant based alternatives fare nutritionally compared to cow's milk?', *Journal of Food Science and Technology* (2018); 55(1): 10–20.

Katz DL, Doughty KN, Geagan K, Jenkins DA, Gardner CD, 'Perspective: The Public Health Case for Modernizing the Definition of Protein Quality', *Advances in Nutrition* (2019); 10(5): 755–64.

Mirzaei, Hamed, *et al.*, 'Protein and amino acid restriction, aging and disease: from yeast to humans', *Trends in Endocrinology and Metabolism* (2014); 25(11): 558–66.

Song, Mingyang, *et al.*, 'Association of Animal and Plant Protein Intake With All-Cause and Cause-Specific Mortality', *JAMA Internal Medicine* (2016); 176(10): 1453–63.

Hahn D, Hodson EM, Fouque D, 'Low protein diets for non-diabetic adults with chronic kidney disease', *Cochrane Database of Systematic Reviews* (2018; 10: CD001892.

Nakamura H, Takasawa M, Kashara S, Tsuda A, Momotsu T, Ito S, Shibata A, 'Effects of acute protein loads of different sources on renal function of patients with diabetic nephropathy', *The Tohoku Journal of Experimental Medicine* (1989); 159(2): 153–62.

Frassetto L.A., Todd K.M., Morris R.C., Sebastian

A., 'Estimation of net endogenous noncarbonic acid production in humans from diet potassium and protein contents', *American Journal of Clinical Nutrition* (1998); 68: 576–83.

Chen, Z., Glisic, M., Song, M., *et al.*, 'Dietary protein intake and all-cause and cause-specific mortality: results from the Rotterdam Study and a meta-analysis of prospective cohort studies', *European Journal of Epidemiology* (2020).

WFPB FOR FAMILIES

Carter JP, Furman T, Hutcheson HR, 'Preeclampsia and reproductive performance in a community of vegans', *Southern Medical Journal* (1987); 80(6): 692–97.

Zhang C, Liu S, Solomon CG, Hu FB, 'Dietary fiber intake, dietary glycemic load, and the risk for gestational diabetes mellitus', *Diabetes Care* (2006); 29(10): 2223–30.

Pistollato F, Sumalla Cano S, Elio I, Masias Vergara M, Giampieri F, Battino M, 'Plant-Based and Plant-Rich Diet Patterns during Gestation: Beneficial Effects and Possible Shortcomings', *Advances in Nutrition* (2015); 6(5): 581–91.

Sebastiani, G., Herranz Barbero, A., Borrás-Novell, C., *et al.*, 'The Effects of Vegetarian and Vegan Diet during Pregnancy on the Health of Mothers and Offspring', *Nutrients* (2019); 11: 557.

Yarrington C, Pearce EN, 'Iodine and pregnancy', *Journal of Thyroid Research* (2011); 2011: 934104.

Cormick G, Belizán JM, 'Calcium Intake and Health', *Nutrients* (2019); 11(7): 1606.

Brannon PM, Taylor CL, 'Iron Supplementation during Pregnancy and Infancy: Uncertainties and Implications for Research and World Health Organization', *Fortification of Food-Grade Salt with Iodine for the Prevention and Control of Iodine Deficiency Disorders* (Geneva, 2014).

Skeaff & Mann, *Essentials of Human Nutrition*, (2012) 4th Edition: Chapter 4: Lipids pp.50–69.

Vandenplas, Yvan, Gutierrez Castrellon, Pedro, Rivas, Rodolfo, *et al.*, 'Systematic Review with Meta-Analysis Safety of soya-based infant formulas in children', *British Journal of Nutrition* (2014); 111: 1340–60.

Kim H, Caulfield LE, Rebholz CM, 'Healthy Plant-Based Diets Are Associated with Lower Risk of All-Cause Mortality in US Adults', *Journal of Nutrition* (2018); 148(4): 624–31.

Alwarith, Jihad, Kahleova, Hana, Crosby, Lee, Brooks, Alexa, Brandon, Lizoralia, Levin, Susan M, Barnard, Neal D, 'The role of nutrition in asthma prevention and treatment', *Nutrition Reviews*.

Haas F, Bishop MC, Salazar-Schicchi J, *et al.*, 'Effect of milk ingestion on pulmonary function in healthy and asthmatic subjects', *Journal of Asthma* (1991); 28: 349–55.

Yusoff NA, Hampton SM, Dickerson JW, *et al.*, 'The effects of exclusion of dietary egg and milk in the management of asthmatic children: a pilot study', *The Journal of the Royal Society for the Promotion of Health* (2004); 124: 74–80.

Nylund L, Nermes M, Isolauri E, Salminen S, de Vos WM, Satokari R, 'Severity of atopic disease inversely correlates with intestinal microbiota diversity and butyrate-producing bacteria', *Allergy* (2015); 70(2): 241–44.

Turner-McGrievy G, Mandes T, Crimarco A, 'A plant-based diet for overweight and obesity prevention and treatment', *Journal of Geriatric Cardiology* (2017); 14(5): 369–74.

Cvejoska-Cholakovska V, Kocova M, Velikj-Stefanovska V, Vlashki E, 'The Association between Asthma and Obesity in Children – Inflammatory and Mechanical Factors', *Open Access Macedonian Journal of Medical Sciences* (2019); 7(8): 1314–19.

Lindahl O, Lindwall L, Spångberg A, *et al.*, 'Vegan regimen with reduced medication in the treatment of bronchial asthma', *Journal of Asthma* (1985); 22: 45–55.

Rice JL, GASP Study Investigators, Romero KM, Galvez Davila RM, *et al.*, 'Association between adherence to the Mediterranean diet and asthma in Peruvian children', *Lung* (2015); 193: 893–99.

Clinton CM, O'Brien S, Law J, Renier CM, Wendt MR, 'Whole-foods, plant-based diet alleviates the symptoms of osteoarthritis', *Arthritis* (2015); 2015: 708152–708161.11.

Min, K., Min, J., 'Association between leukocyte telomere length and serum carotenoid in US adults', *European Journal of Nutrition* (2017); 56: 1045–52.

Drewnowski A, Shultz JM, 'Impact of aging on eating behaviors, food choices, nutrition, and health status', *The Journal of Nutrition, Health and Aging* (2001); 5(2): 75–9.

Lonnie M, Hooker E, Brunstrom JM, *et al.*, 'Protein for Life: Review of Optimal Protein Intake, Sustainable Dietary Sources and the Effect on Appetite in Ageing Adults', *Nutrients* (2018); 10(3): 360.

Rejnmark L, 'Effects of vitamin d on muscle function and performance: a review of evidence from randomized controlled trials', *Therapeutic Advances in Chronic Disease* (2011); 2(1): 25–37.

Dhesi JK, Bearne LM, Moniz C, *et al.*, 'Neuromuscular and psychomotor function in elderly subjects who fall and the relationship with vitamin D status', *Journal of Bone and Mineral Research* (2002); 17(5): 891–97.

Halfon M, Phan O, Teta D, 'Vitamin D: a review on its effects on muscle strength, the risk of fall, and frailty', *BioMed Research International* (2015); 2015: 953241.

Lam JR, Schneider JL, Zhao W, Corley DA, 'Proton pump inhibitor and histamine 2 receptor antagonist use and vitamin B12 deficiency', *JAMA* (2013); 310(22): 2435–42.

SUPPLEMENTS

Lehotský J, Tothová B, Kovalská M, *et al.*, 'Role of Homocysteine in the Ischemic Stroke and Development of Ischemic Tolerance', *Frontiers in Neuroscience* (2016); 10: 538. doi: 10.3389/fnins.2016.00538.

Paul C, Brady DM, 'Comparative Bioavailability and Utilization of Particular Forms of B12 Supplements With Potential to Mitigate B12-related Genetic Polymorphisms', *Integrative Medicine (Encinitas)* (2017); 16(1): 42–9.

Rodriguez-Leyva D, Weighell W, Edel AL, *et al.*, 'Potent antihypertensive action of dietary flaxseed in hypertensive patients', *Hypertension* (2013); 62(6): 1081–89.

Caligiuri SP, Aukema HM, Ravandi A, Guzman R, Dibrov E, Pierce GN, 'Flaxseed consumption reduces blood pressure in patients with hypertension by altering circulating oxylipins via an α-linolenic acid-induced inhibition of soluble epoxide hydrolase', *Hypertension* (2014); 64(1): 53–9.

Caligiuri SP, Rodriguez-Leyva D, Aukema HM, *et al.*, 'Dietary Flaxseed Reduces Central Aortic Blood Pressure Without Cardiac Involvement but Through Changes in Plasma Oxylipins', *Hypertension* (2016); 68(4): 1031–38. doi: 10.1161/HYPERTENSIONAHA.116.07834

A NEW WAY TO EAT

Wansink, Brian & Sobal, Jeffery, 'Mindless Eating: The 200 Daily Food Decisions We Overlook', *Environemnt and Behavior* (2007); 39: 106–23.

Mann, Traci, *Secrets from the Eating Lab: The*

Science of Weight Loss, the Myth of Willpower and Why You Should Never Diet Again (Harper Wave 2017).

CONCLUSION

Carroll D, Watson B, Togami E, *et al*., 'Building a global atlas of zoonotic viruses', *Bulletin of the World Health Organization* (2018); 96(4): 292–94.

Taubenberger JK, 'The origin and virulence of the 1918 "Spanish" influenza virus', *Proceedings of the American Philosophy Society* (2006); 150(1): 86–112.

Kandeil A, Gomaa M, Nageh A, *et al*., 'Middle East Respiratory Syndrome Coronavirus (MERS-CoV) in Dromedary Camels in Africa and Middle East', *Viruses* (2019); 11(8): 717.

Wang LF, Eaton BT, 'Bats, civets and the emergence of SARS', *Current Topics in Microbiol ogy and Immunology* (2007); 315: 325–44.

Zhang T, Wu Q, Zhang Z, 'Probable Pangolin Origin of SARS-CoV-2 Associated with the COVID-19 Outbreak', *Current Biology* (2020); 30(7): 1346–1351.e2. [published correction appears in *Current Biology* (2020); 30(8): 1578]

Gebreyes WA, Dupouy-Camet J, Newport MJ, *et al*., 'The global one health paradigm: challenges and opportunities for tackling infectious diseases at the human, animal, and environment interface in low-resource settings', *PLOS Neglected Tropical Diseases* (2014); 8(11): e3257.

Founou LL, Founou RC, Essack SY, 'Antibiotic Resistance in the Food Chain: A Developing Country-Perspective', *Frontiers in Microbiology* (2016); 7: 1881.

Heredia N, García S, 'Animals as sources of food-borne pathogens: A review', *Animal Nutrition* (2018); 4(3): 250–55.

Dinu, Monica, Abbate, Rosanna, Gensini, Gianfranco, Casini, Alessandro, Sofi, Francesco, 'Vegetarian, vegan diets and multiple health outcomes: A systematic review with meta-analysis with meta-analysis of observational studies', *Critical Reviews in Food Science and Nutrition* (2017) 57: 3640–49.

'2019 ACC/AHA Guideline on the Primary Prevention of Cardiovascular Disease: A Report of the American College of Cardiology/American Heart Association Task Force on Clinical Practice Guidelines', *Journal of the American College of Cardiology* (2019).

Kelly, J., Karlsen, M.,Steinke, G., 'Type 2 Diabetes Remission and Lifestyle Medicine: A Position Statement From the American College of Lifestyle Medicine', *American Journal of Lifestyle Medicine* (2020).

Steffen W, Persson A, Deutsch L, *et al*., 'The anthropocene: from global change to planetary stewardship', *AMBIO* (2011); 40(7): 739–61.

Razis DV, 'The risk of a sixth mass extinction of life and the role of medicine', *Journal of the Royal Society of Medicine* (2010); 103(12): 473–74.

Ceballos G, Ehrlich PR, Barnosky AD, García A, Pringle RM, Palmer TM, 'Accelerated modern human-induced species losses: Entering the sixth mass extinction', *Science Advances* (2015); 1(5): e1400253.

Bowles DC, Butler CD, Morisetti N, 'Climate change, conflict and health. *Journal of the Royal Society of Medicine*', (2015); 108(10): 390–95.

FURTHER READING

BOOKS

Robby Barbaro and Cyrus Khambatta, *Mastering Diabetes* (Penguin Random House USA, 2020)

Brené Brown, *Daring Greatly* (Penguin Life, 2015)

Dr Rangan Chatterjee, *The Stress Solution* (Penguin Life, 2018)

Garth Davis M.D., *Proteinaholic* (HarperOne, 2016)

Jonathan Safran Foer, *Eating Animals* (Penguin, 2011)

Jonathan Safran Foer, *We are the Weather* (Hamish Hamilton, 2019)

BJ Fogg, *Tiny Habits* (Virgin Books, 2019)

Dr Michael Greger, *How Not To Die* (Pan, 2017)

Rich Roll, *Finding Ultra* (Three Rivers Press, 2013)

FILMS

Forks Over Knives, Lee Fulkerson (dir), (Monica Beach Media, 2011)

The Game Changers, Louie Psihoyos (dir), (Fathom Events, 2019)

WEBSITES

www.gemmanewman.com where you will find a plethora of information as well as all the references used in the compilation of this book.

www.plantbasedhealthprofessionals.com where you will find information leaflets, online courses and blogs on the benefits of plant-based nutrition.

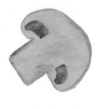

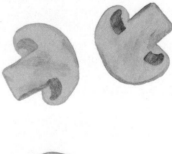

INDEX

RECIPE INDEX

MEAL PLANNERS

	BREAKFAST	LUNCH	DINNER	DESSERT	SNACKS
MONDAY					
TUESDAY					
WEDNESDAY					
THURSDAY					
FRIDAY					
SATURDAY					
SUNDAY					

THE PLANT POWER DOCTOR

	BREAKFAST	LUNCH	DINNER	DESSERT	SNACKS
MONDAY					
TUESDAY					
WEDNESDAY					
THURSDAY					
FRIDAY					
SATURDAY					
SUNDAY					

NOTES

THE PLANT POWER DOCTOR

ACKNOWLEDGEMENTS

All my gratitude goes to every single person who made this book possible, and I thank you from the bottom of my heart for the passion, guidance and perseverance it took from each of you to turn dreams into reality.

Thank you to Richard Newman, my soulmate and first editor. Thank you for your deep love, intelligence and support every step of the way. Thank you to my friend Georgina Rodgers, whose astute perspective, time management and talents took this book where it needed to go. Thank you to Laura for believing in me every step of the way, Catherine Phipps for your skills with recipe development and Dave Brown, Becky and Dan for bringing the recipes (and me!) to life. Thank you Sjaniel Turrell for your kindness and skills. Dave thank you also for your amazing creativity with book design. Carmen – thank you for your beautiful illustrations, both in my book and on my website, which have truly brought my mission to life. Thank you also to Rob and Carol at MAD Ideas for your talents, kindness and ethos. Thank you to Sam and everyone else at Ebury, Penguin Random House for your support, it has meant the world to me. Thank you to Rowan Lawton, you are the best agent I could wish for.

There are others to whom I also owe great debt in writing this book. Thank you to the incredible dietician, nutritionist, international speaker and author Brenda Davis, for your generous mentorship and commentary on my first drafts. Thank you to nutritionist Rohini Bajekal for your thorough guidance and help. Your friendship and support mean so much to me. Thank you also to dietician Rosie Martin and nutritionist Prabha Shiyani for your helpful feedback. Thank you to the amazing chef Day Radley for your recipe support. Thank you to Dr Shireen Kassam for your support and all you do at PBHPUK. Thank you to the inimitable David and Stephen Flynn for your energy, enthusiasm and light. Thank you to Ayan Panja for reminding me GPs can save lives in slow motion, Rangan Chatterjee for your guidance and Rupy Aujla for your inspirational example.

Thank you to Dr Cyrus Khambatta for allowing me to include your story as a case study, as well as for yours and Robbie Barbaro's unwavering support. Thank you to Dr Em Deacon for your inspiring story and incredible heart. Thank you to Dr Saray Stancic, Dr Brooke Goldner, Dr Conor Kerley, and friends Iida van der Byl Knoefel and Brendan Kelly for being inspirational examples of the power of the plate to heal disease. Thank you to all of my patients who inspire me, ground me and teach me every day in clinic. It is a privilege and an honour. Thank you for allowing me glimpses into your life, and letting me share in the joys and tragedies you face. I will never take it for granted.

Thank you to my professional hero Dr Neal Barnard, founder of The Physicians Committee for Responsible Medicine, for your tireless contribution to medical research. Thank you to Rich Roll and to Srimati for your unparalleled wisdom and generosity. You have both given the world more than you can imagine, through the power of peace, plants and connection.

Thank you to Vicky Miles, everybody needs a Vicky! Thank you to my close friends who have supported me always, you know who you are. Thank you to my work colleagues and partner Miriam, you all make my job infinitely more special with your kindness and support. Thank you to my family. Especially my sister (the first vegan I ever met) and my mum for your unconditional love. Thank you to my boys Max and Ted. You inspire me to be a better person every day and teach me so much.

Lastly, thank you to each and every person who decided to pick up this book and take it home. You have made it all worthwhile.

DISCLAIMER

For some of us, lifestyle choices are optimal when personalised to us – our pre-existing medical conditions, our bio-individuality, our medications and our history.

Even though I am a medical doctor, this book is really for education and inspiration. Speak to your own doctor, dietician or nutritionist if you have a medical condition. The information in this book is not meant as a replacement for medical treatment and is not medical advice. Positive lifestyle changes act alongside any medical intervention and in some cases may mean pills and procedures are not needed. But this is not always the case and so it is crucial that you seek advice from your own doctor if you have a medical condition.

Some nutritionists and dieticians have seen people in their clinics who have a tendency towards dietary restriction because their clients have focused on what they feel they should be eating, or controlling what they can't have. Some of them may even have adopted veganism as part of this pattern. This can be very difficult psychologically. When you have specific medical and psychological needs that require you to receive advice from a registered nutritionist or trained dietician, a book like this can quite simply never replace their advice.

The data included in this book is from a variety of reputable sources; from researchers, doctors and journal articles, large population trials, randomised controlled trials, laboratory studies and international guidelines. Wherever possible, I will explain where information has come from within the text, and some of the key references are available on pages 268–90. There are nearly 600 references cited in total, and all references for you to check are included on my website. They are listed sentence by sentence so you can see exactly where they are. I want for you to understand that the information I share has been observed and studied in the scientific literature. I also use case studies from my own experience to bring the text to life in a way that facts and figures could never do. Good nutrition can save lives. Holistic approaches to health can change the stories of heartache for thousands of families across the globe. This is why I include some real people in order for this to feel real to you too. I would love for you to feel empowered to make the changes you want to see in your life, as many of my patients have.

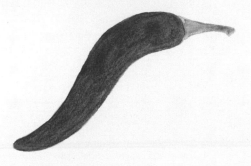

1

Published in 2021 by Ebury Press an imprint of Ebury Publishing,
20 Vauxhall Bridge Road,
London SW1V 2SA

Ebury Press is part of the Penguin Random House group of companies whose addresses can be found at global.penguinrandomhouse.com

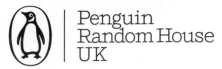

Penguin
Random House
UK

First published by Ebury Press in 2021

www.penguin.co.uk

A CIP catalogue record for this book is available from the British Library

ISBN 9781529107746

Text design: Ape Inc. Ltd
Photography: Dave Brown except page 9 from Jeremie Dupont, and pages 2, 7, 29, 38, 51, 62, 78, 97, 111, 123, 131, 168, and 185 from Getty Images
Food styling: Rebecca Woods
Prop styling: Olivia Wardle
Watercolours: Carmen Wan-Easterby at Mad Ideas
Colour reproduction: Altaimage Ltd
Printed and bound in Italy by L.E.G.O. S.p.A

The authorised representative in the EEA is Penguin Random House Ireland, Morrison Chambers, 32 Nassau Street, Dublin D02 YH68.

Penguin Random House is committed to a sustainable future for our business, our readers and our planet. This book is made from Forest Stewardship Council® certified paper.

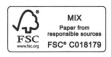